THE CBD HANDBOOK

OVER 75 RECIPES
for Hemp-Derived Health and Wellness

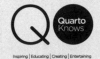

Brimming with creative inspiration, how-to projects, and useful information to enrich your everyday life, Quarto Knows is a favorite destination for those pursuing their interests and passions. Visit our site and dig deeper with our books into your area of interest: Quarto Creates, Quarto Cooks, Quarto Homes, Quarto Lives, Quarto Drives, Quarto Explores, Quarto Gifts, or Quarto Kids.

First published in 2019 by Chartwell Books,
an imprint of The Quarto Group,
142 West 36th Street, 4th Floor
New York, NY 10018, USA
T (212) 779-4972 F (212) 779-6058
www.QuartoKnows.com

Chartwell titles are also available at discount for retail, wholesale, promotional and bulk purchase. For details, contact the Special Sales Manager by email at specialsales@quarto.com or by mail at The Quarto Group, Attn: Special Sales Manager, 100 Cummings Center Suite, 265D, Beverly, MA 01915, USA.

The publisher cannot guarantee the accuracy, adequacy, or completeness of the information contained in this book and must disclaim all warranties, expressed or implied, regarding the information. The publisher also cannot assume any responsibility for use of this book, and any use by a reader is at the reader's own risk. This book is not intended to be a substitute for professional medical advice, and any user of this book should always check with a licensed physician before adopting any particular course of treatment or beginning any new health program.

ISBN: 978-0-7858-3786-2

Library of Congress Control Number: 2019945928

10 9 8 7 6 5 4 3 2 1

Publisher: Rage Kindelsperger
Creative Director: Laura Drew
Managing Editor: Cara Donaldson
Editor: Leeann Moreau
Cover and Page Design: Amy Harte for 3&Co.

THE CBD HANDBOOK

OVER 75 RECIPES
for Hemp-Derived Health and Wellness

Melissa Petitto, R.D.

CHARTWELL
BOOKS

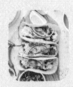

DRINKS 47

CBD-Infused
Rum Thai Iced Tea
49

Coconut Matcha
CBD Tea Latte
51

Fruity Party Vodka
CBD Punch
52

Mint & Watermelon
CBD Mojito
53

CBD Ginger-Turmeric
Golden Milk
54

Mocha
Oat CBD Latte
55

The Updated
Margarita
57

CBD Period Relief Tea
Latte
59

Calming Berry Vanilla
CBD Smoothie
60

Green Recovery
CBD Smoothie
61

MAINS 63

Baby Kale, Orange,
Walnuts & Olive Salad
w/ Citrus Vinaigrette
65

Shrimp Summer
Rolls w/ Sweet
Chili Sauce
66

Watermelon & Tomato
Gazpacho w/ CBD
Olive Oil Drizzle
69

Chana Saag Chickpea
Spinach Curry with
Crispy CBD Chickpeas
70

Escarole & White
Bean Soup w/ CBD
Infused Broth
73

Green Mango Mung Bean
Noodle Salad w/ CBD Toasted
Coconut Grilled Shrimp
75

Tomato, Watermelon,
Basil & Arugula Salad with
CBD Balsamic Dressing
77

The Ultimate Vegan
—or Not—Grilled
Cheese
79

Italian Stuffed Artichokes
w/ CBD-Infused Lemon
Sauce
81

Fish Tacos
with Cabbage &
Radishes
83

Miso, Yam, Carrot,
& Ginger CBD
Recovery Soup
85

CBD-infused
Pasta
Margarita
87

Spaghetti with
CBD Pistachio
Pesto
89

Falafel with
Garlicky CBD
Tahini Sauce
90

Ground Chicken/Vegetable
Protein Laarb w/ Mint & Thai
Basil in Lettuce Cups
93

SIDE DISHES

CBD
Quinoa
Tabbouleh
97

Easy "Creamed" Corn
w/ Thyme, Rosemary
& CBD
99

Grilled & Smashed
New Potatoes w/ CBD
Crème Fraîche
101

Grilled Vegetables
with Green Tahini Sauce
103

Spinach-Artichoke
Gratin w/ CBD
104

Braised Winter Greens
w/ Black Garlic & CBD
107

Roasted Ginger Carrots w/
CBD Miso Sauce
109

PET SNACKS

Bacon-Sweet Potato
CBD Treats
112

Sweet Potato & Salmon
CBD Cat Treats
115

Mackerel & Coconut
CBD Cat Treats
116

Tuna CBD Thumbprint
Cat Treats
117

Baby Food
CBD Dog Treats
119

Ginger-Apple
CBD
Bones
121

CBD Honey &
Peanut Butter
Dog Biscuits
123

Coconut & Turmeric
CBD Breath
Mints
124

Frozen Peanut
Butter
Yogurt Treats
125

No-Bake Coconut
Oat Ball
Dog Treats
127

SELF-CARE 129

INTRODUCTION

CBD*, or Cannabidiol, is widely used for many ailments:

- pain relief
- reducing inflammation
- controlling anxiety and depression
- reducing acne breakouts
- alleviating cancer-related symptoms
- improving heart health
- helping with smoking cessation and drug withdrawal
- reducing the effects of chronic pain multiple sclerosis, and arthritis pain
- aiding in the treatment of seizures and epilepsy, and possibly helping with type 1 diabetes

As you can see, the use for CBD varies greatly, and we have only just scratched the surface of what this powerful compound can do. (Jillian Kubala, 2018)

You may be asking, "How will my body feel when I start taking CBD?" There is no "high feeling" or psychoactive effects from CBD, although some people can feel a bit drowsy. One of the most amazing qualities of CBD is its chameleon-like properties. Research has found that depending on what ails you, whether inflammation or anxiety, CBD can help aid in reducing the effects and treating symptoms of an illness.

Of course, everyone is different and therefore should check with a doctor before introducing CBD into their health regimens. When including CBD into your daily routine, most people sleep better, feel less stressed out, report less soreness and inflammation in their muscles, and are able to focus better.

*The FDA has not released a ruling yet on CBD; however, the FDA does consider it safe for consumption.

FORMS OF CBD

Cannabinoids are compounds found in the cannabis plant. There are hundreds of cannabinoids in the cannabis plant, of which CBD and THC are two of the most naturally occurring compounds. In 1995 research uncovered that CBD can deliver unique health benefits within the body. (Cadena, Gill, 2018) While THC is responsible for the majority of the psychoactive effects of the cannabis plant, CBD counteracts these effects.

CBD to be ingested comes in four main forms: (1) CBD isolate/crystals, (2) full-spectrum oil, (3) broad-spectrum oil, and (4) water-soluble CBD. These four forms are extremely different. Here's how to choose which one you want to use and how to use them. (Foria, 2018)

CBD Isolate/Crystals

An isolate is the purest form of a compound. When CBD isolate is produced, all other compounds found in the cannabis plant, including terpenes, flavonoids, and other cannabinoids, are removed. The hemp plant is what is traditionally used for isolate because of its low to non-existent THC content. CBD isolate is used by a lot of companies and our bodies do not know how to metabolize isolate, so it is best for external use. Its benefits include:

- **purest form of CBD**
- **tasteless and odorless**
- **no THC**
- **does not deliver the "entourage effect," no enhanced benefits**

Full-Spectrum CBD Oil

Full-spectrum CBD oil contains all of the compounds found naturally in the plant, including terpenes, essential oils, and other cannabinoids, and this creates the "entourage effect." The "entourage effect" occurs in full-spectrum CBD, since all of these naturally occurring compounds work together to magnify the therapeutic benefits of each individual cannabinoid. Full-spectrum CBD can have trace amounts of THC, but it is intentionally left so that it can activate more of the beneficial effects of CBD. In 2005, scientists found that full-spectrum CBD oil provided higher levels of pain and stress relief than CBD isolate. (Cadena, 2018) Its benefits include:

- **the "entourage effect"**
- **less processed than other forms**
- **may show up on drug tests**
- **may contain small traces of THC**
- **may have a stronger natural flavor**
- **may have sedative effects**

Broad-Spectrum CBD Oil

This form of CBD is a blend of full-spectrum and isolate. Like CBD isolate, the THC is completely removed, but, like full-spectrum, he other compounds within the plant are preserved. Its benefits include:

- the "entourage effect"
- no THC
- more processed
- may have a stronger natural flavor
- less research readily available
- processed to remove THC from final product

Water-Soluble CBD

This form of CBD takes quite a bit of help from science. As mentioned above, CBD needs a fat as a carrier to be absorbed into the body. With a little help, water-soluble CBD is formulated to be water compatible. (Corren, 2018) This form is wonderful for use in cocktails, teas, coffees, and other beverages. Its benefits include:

- fast-acting, typically 30 seconds compared to 30 minutes with CBD oil delivery
- claims to be the most bioavailable
- usually a lower mg content per bottle

INDEPENDENT THIRD-PARTY TESTING

The CBD industry is not currently regulated by the FDA; therefore, having an independent third-party lab test CBD products allows a neutral, unbiased source examine the quality and content of a company's product. I always suggest buying a third-party tested CBD product. This is just one way to ensure you are purchasing a quality product and that the company is not scared to have an outside source verify it. Don't be afraid to reach out to the CBD companies that you're investigating. They should be able to provide you with a Certificate of Analysis (COA) to tell you exactly what is in the specific batch of CBD oil that you're purchasing. If they don't respond to you, feel free to try another company. (Gill, 2018)

I asked the owner of Saving Grace CBD. His products are my go-to, and this is what he said:

- full-spectrum is recommended, but if you're sensitive to THC, try one of the others
- always buy CO^2 extracted
- new technology is coming out rapidly since the farm bill has been passed, so the industry is changing
- do not shop by the cost per bottle, shop by the cost per mg

DOSAGE AND HEALTH CONCERNS

CBD is incredibly individualized. What works for one person might not work perfectly for another. It is always recommended to start with a low dosage and increase as needed. An increase after two weeks is optimal. A general guideline for dosing includes:

- **for general health: 2.5 to 15 mg CBD per day**
- **for chronic pain: 2.5 to 100 mg CBD per day**
- **for sleep issues: 40 to 175 mg CBD per day**

Body weight is also an important factor to determine how much CBD you require. A good rule of thumb is 1 to 6 mg of CBD for every 10 pounds (4.5 kg) of body weight. (Pure Kana, 2018)

Keeping track of how much CBD you take per day, for how long, and at what time is a great way to learn how various doses work for you. Below is a simple chart illustrating CBD dosages based on your weight and level of physical discomfort.

DOSAGE BY BODY WEIGHT

LEVEL OF PAIN	<25 lbs	26-45 lbs	46-85 lbs	86-150 lbs	151-240 lbs	>241 lbs
None-Mild	4.5 mg	6 mg	9 mg	12 mg	18 mg	22.5 mg
Medium	6 mg	9 mg	12 mg	15 mg	22.5 mg	30 mg
Severe	9 mg	12 mg	15 mg	18 mg	27 mg	45 mg

Each consumable recipe is labeled with low, medium, and high dose symbols:

 LOW 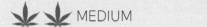 MEDIUM 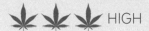 HIGH

Since it is best to start low and work your way up, the mg content in our grading system skews low. Worried about taking too much CBD? Studies have shown that in order for CBD to be toxic in the body, you would have to ingest almost 20,000 mg of CBD oil in a very short period of time. If you happen to take too much for your own body, you might feel the need for a nap. Other studies have found that too much CBD may cause diarrhea, changes in appetite, and fatigue. (CBD Oil Review, n.d.)

Choosing the right CBD oil for yourself can be overwhelming, but luckily the website CBD Oil Review (cbdoilreview.org) breaks down CBD companies and helps readers choose the right one. As mentioned previously, the FDA does not currently regulate CBD, so researching on your own is necessary.

There are countless variables such as weight, diet, metabolism, genetics, environment, and product consistency that makes a universal dosage impossible to calculate. I, for example, take CBD full-spectrum oil for anxiety and to aid with sleep. I weigh 115 pounds and take 55 mg to 75 mg a day. I have athlete friends who take it for muscle recovery and take upwards of 100 mg a day.

The best advice is to start low, keep a journal of how it makes you feel, and increase slowly until YOU find the right dosage for YOURSELF. Another component to keep in mind when ingesting CBD is that it is processed by the liver and other digestive organs. This means that only a small percentage makes it into the bloodstream to be used by the endocannabinoid system. The excess is stored in fat cells and is gradually released for days afterwards. This is why it is so important to consume CBD consistently to see the benefits.

Vita Leaf Naturals (https://vitaleafnaturals.com) has a CBD dosage calculator that I find quite helpful in finding the CBD dose that's right for me. Other favorite websites for all your CBD needs include:

- **https://www.projectcbd.org/**
- **https://www.green-flower.com/**
- **https://www.medicaljane.com/**

COOKING WITH CBD

In this book, I mostly use full-spectrum CBD oil. CBD is fat soluble, which means that consuming it with a healthy dose of fats can increase the amount of CBD that is absorbed by the bloodstream—in addition, more cannabinoids are absorbed on a full stomach.

APPROXIMATE DOSE PER DROP

BASED ON A 30ML CONTAINER	DROP	.25 ml	.5 ml	1 ml
200 mg	⅓ mg	1¾ mg	3½ mg	7 mg
300 mg	⅕ mg	2½ mg	5 mg	10 mg
500 mg	⅘ mg	4¼ mg	8½ mg	17 mg
600 mg	1 mg	5 mg	10 mg	20 mg
800 mg	1⅓ mg	6¾ mg	13½ mg	27 mg
1000 mg	1⅔ mg	8¾ mg	17½ mg	35 mg
1200 mg	2 mg	10 mg	20 mg	40 mg
1500 mg	2½ mg	12½ mg	25 mg	50 mg

Before you can cook with CBD, it is best to infuse it into a fat- or oil-based product, such as coconut oil, butter, or ghee. CBD infused coconut oil can nowbe found in most health food stores. In some recipes, alcohol can replace the fat component, unless you are using water-soluble CBD. Wine and beer are not good carriers for CBD oil because they are water based.

You will notice in this book that I never heat CBD oil over high heat. This is because cannabinoids evaporate, thus losing their potency when they come into contact with high heat. The boiling point for cannabidiol is between 320°F and 365°F (160°C to 185°C). You will often see that I add CBD to a recipe after it comes off the heat or only heat it over low to medium heat. This is incredibly important to keep in mind!

PET SNACKS

CBD greatly affects household pets in a similar way to how it affects humans. Nervous animals can be difficult to handle, whether it's because of a specific stressor (such as, they don't like the car) or they are generally a little neurotic.

A dose of CBD can calm our furry friends just as it calms us. For older arthritic animals, CBD can also be away to help your pets with pain management. Consult with your vet before adding CBD treats to your pet's diet.

Basic dosing rule for cats and dogs: 1-5 mg CBD for every 10 pounds of body weight. They may be given a dose every 8 hours for pain and anxiety management.

SELF-CARE

Bath bombs, lip balms, toners, and scrubs! CBD is a great way to topically soothe irritation. You will notice that the amount of CBD in our self-care section is much higher than when you ingest it orally. When applied topically, a generous application is recommended for optimal results. Topical CBD disperses across your skin and is localized to its targets, like sore muscles, inflammation, and pain perceiving nerves. Very little actually enters the bloodstream when applied this way.

Bibliography

Cadena, Aaron. 2017. *Full-spectrum vs. Broad Spectrum vs. CBD Isolate; The Difference Explained, February, 2017*

CBD Oil Review. n.d. *CBD Oil Dosage: General Tips to Assess How Much CBD to Take.*
https://cbdoilreview.org/cbd-cannabidiol/cbd-dosage/.

Corren, Alex. 2018. *Water-Soluble vs. Oil-Soluble CBD : What You Need To Know.* February 20.
https://uncannywellness.com/blogs/blogs/water-soluble-vs-oil-soluble-cbd-what-you-need-to-know.

Foria. 2018. *How to Take Your CBD.* August 1.
https://www.foriawellness.com/blogs/learn/how-to-take-cbd-correct-dose.

Gill, Lisa L. 2018. *How to Shop for CBD.* September 27.
https://www.consumerreports.org/cbd/how-to-shop-for-cbd/.

Jillian Kubala, MS, RD. 2018. *7 Benefits and Uses of CBD Oil (Plus Side Effects).* February 2018.
https://www.healthline.com/nutrition/cbd-oil-benefits#section2.

Pure Kana. 2018. *HOW TO TAKE CBD [GENERAL DOSAGE GUIDE].* December 25.
https://purekana.com/blogs/news/how-to-take-cbd-general-dosage-guide/.

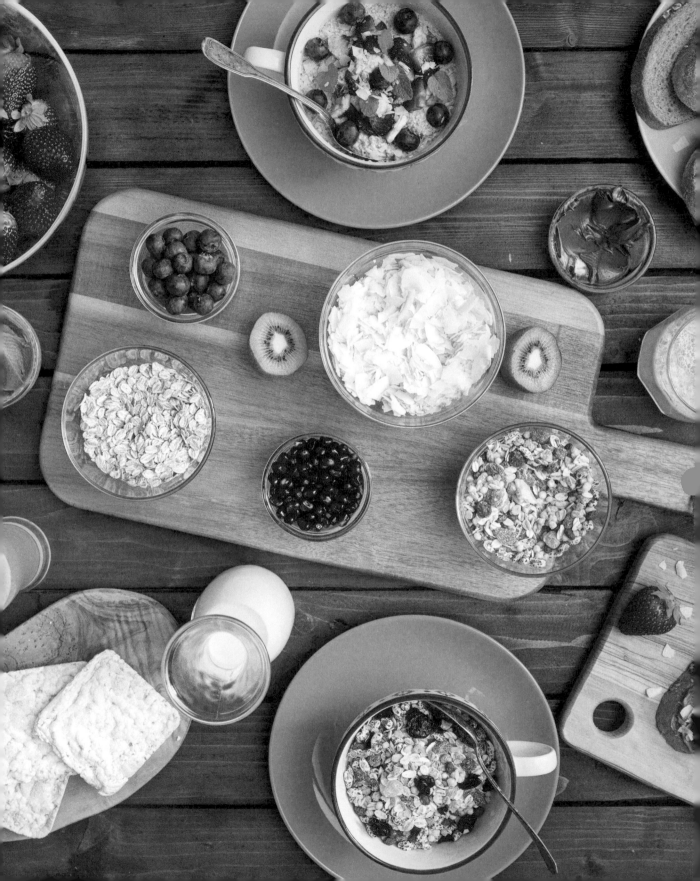

BREAKFAST

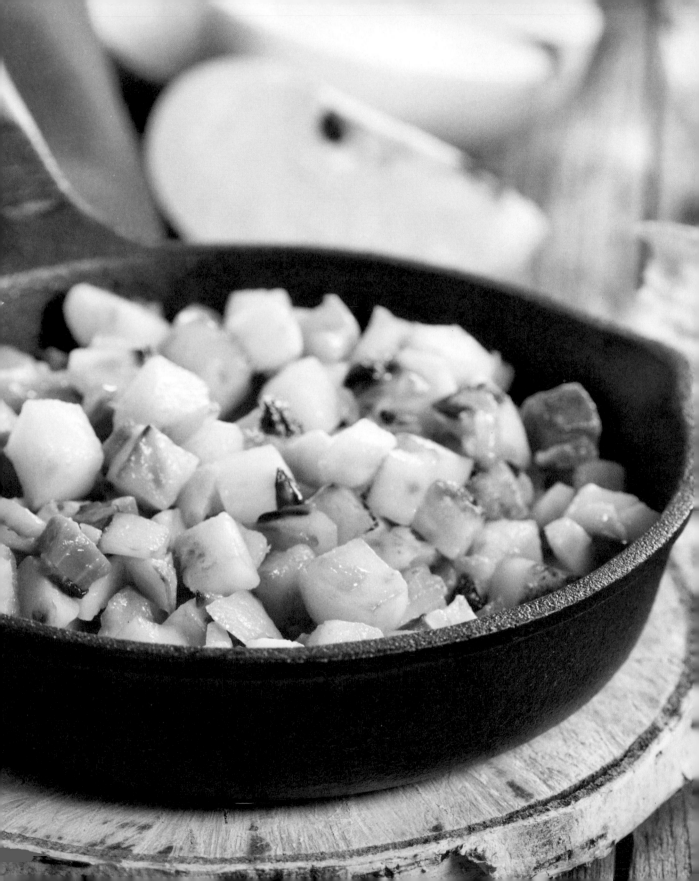

CALMING CBD
BREAKFAST POTATOES

Yield: Serves 6 / about 5 mg per serving

These breakfast potatoes are so tasty and have the added benefit of giving you a low dosage of CBD to calmly start your day.

INGREDIENTS

For the potatoes:
2 pounds (908 g) russet potatoes, washed, peeled, and diced into ½-inch (1 cm) cubes
3 tablespoons (45 ml) avocado oil
1 teaspoon kosher salt
½ teaspoon garlic powder
½ teaspoon paprika
½ teaspoon onion powder
¼ teaspoon freshly ground black pepper
2 tablespoons (28 g) CBD-infused coconut oil
1 sweet onion, chopped
1 green bell pepper, seeded and chopped

TIP *Make sure you have fresh spices; they are the pizazz in this recipe. Ground spices typically only stay fresh for 1-3 years after opening.*

METHOD OF PREPARATION:

1. Preheat the oven to 400°F (200°C). Line a large baking sheet with a silicone baking mat and set aside.

2. In a large bowl, combine the potatoes, avocado oil, salt, garlic powder, paprika, onion powder, and pepper. Toss well to coat.

3. Transfer the spiced potatoes to the prepared baking sheet and arrange in a single layer. Bake for 20 to 25 minutes, or until softened and beginning to brown.

4. While the potatoes bake, in a large skillet heat over medium-low heat, melt the CBD-infused coconut oil.

5. Add the onion and green bell pepper and sauté for 10 to 15 minutes, or until softened and translucent. Do not turn the heat up; this will deactivate the CBD.

6. Once the potatoes are done roasting, turn the oven to broil. Broil the potatoes for 4 to 5 minutes until golden brown and crispy.

7. Add the potatoes to the CBD onions and peppers and toss to coat. Check for seasoning and serve!

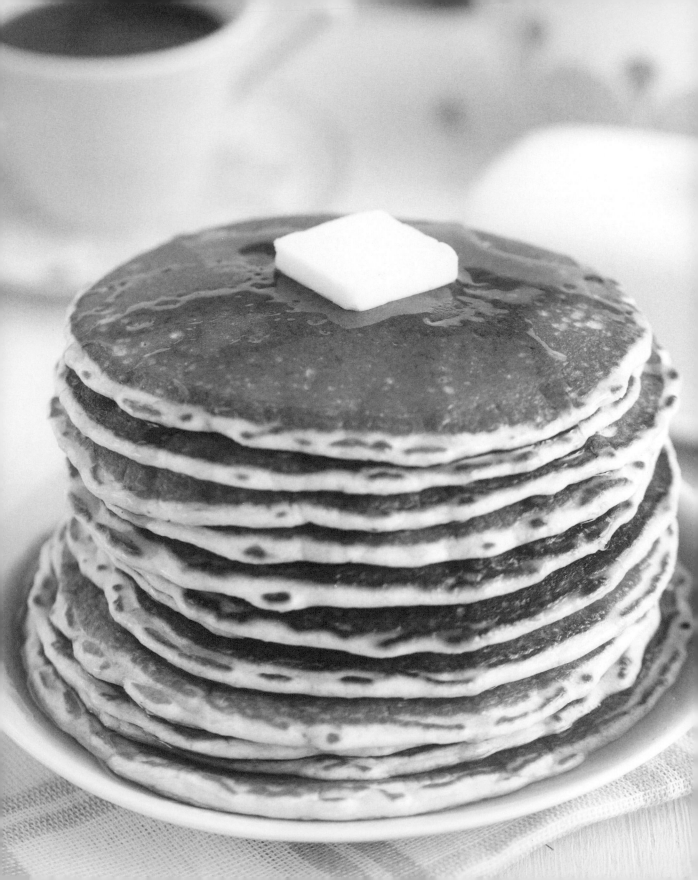

CBD-INFUSED
LIGHT & FLUFFY PANCAKES

Yield: Serves 6, makes 12 pancakes / 5 mg CBD per serving

These pancakes are just the perfect weekend breakfast! With a moderate amount of CBD, you could have them to start a relaxing day or to aid in an intense workout.

INGREDIENTS

2 cups (248 g) unbleached all-purpose flour
¼ cup (38 g) coconut sugar
4 teaspoons (18.5 g) baking powder
½ teaspoon sea salt
¼ teaspoon baking soda
1½ to 1¾ cups (360 to 420 ml) hemp milk, plus more as needed
4 tablespoons (56 g) butter or dairy-free butter such as Miyoko's, melted and cooled slightly
1 teaspoon vanilla extract
1 large egg or 3 tablespoons (45 ml) aquafaba*
30 mg full-spectrum CBD oil
Pure maple syrup, for serving

* Aquafaba is the liquid from a can of chickpeas and it is an incredible substitute for eggs!

METHOD OF PREPARATION:

1. In a large bowl, combine the flour, coconut sugar, baking powder, salt, and baking soda. Whisk well. Make a well in the center of the dry ingredients and add the milk, melted butter, vanilla, and egg. Whisk the wet ingredients in the well and then use a rubber spatula to slowly fold the wet ingredients into the dry ingredients. Before the mixture is completely combined, add the CBD oil and finish mixing. It's okay if there are a few lumps (the batter will be thick and creamy in consistency). If it's too thick, fold in 2 tablespoons (30 ml) of milk. The batter should pour off a ladle smoothly.

2. Set the batter aside and let rest while heating your pan or griddle.

3. Heat a nonstick skillet or griddle over medium-low heat and spray it with a little nonstick cooking spray. Pour ¼ cup (28 g) of the batter into the pan and gently spread it out with the back of a ladle.

4. Pour ¼ cup (28 g) of the batter into the pan and gently spread it out with the back of a ladle. Cook until the underside is golden, and bubbles begin to appear on the surface, about 3 to 4 minutes. Flip with a spatula and cook until golden on the other side, about 3 minutes more. Repeat with remaining pancake batter, keeping the cooked pancakes warm as you go.

5. Serve with maple syrup.

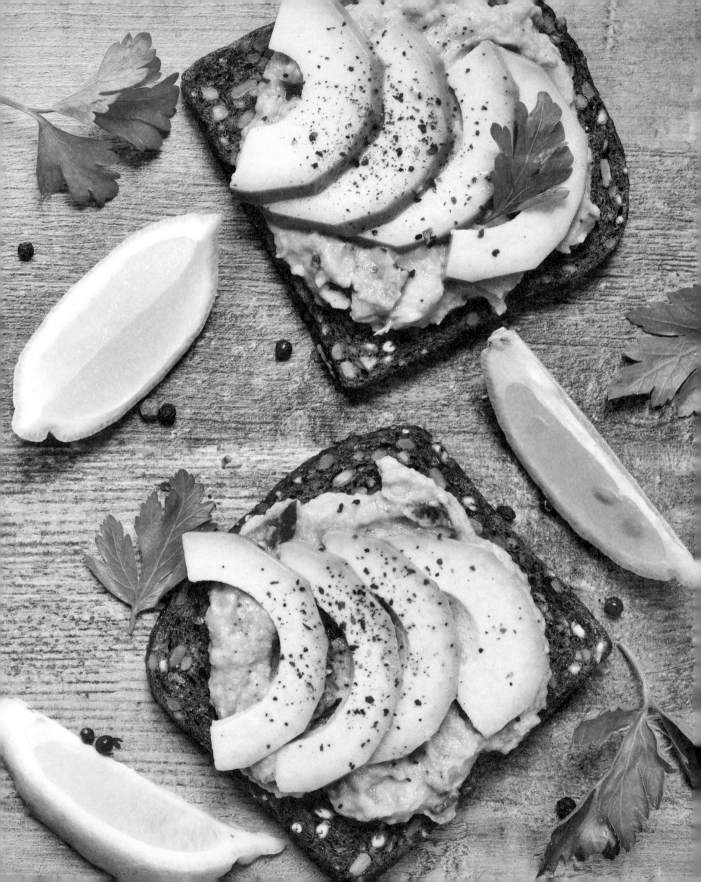

CBD AVOCADO TOAST
WITH SAUERKRAUT, SEA SALT & LEMON ZEST

Yield: Serves 2 / 4 to 5 mg per serving

Avocado toast is so popular right now and rightly so...it's such a nutritious and delicious start to the day. I've jazzed up the normal one, topping it with some probiotic sauerkraut and tangy lemon zest. This one is low on the CBD dosage.

INGREDIENTS

2 slices artisan-quality, thick-sliced, whole-wheat pumpernickle bread or other favorite bread

1 large ripe avocado, peeled and pitted

8 to 10 mg full-spectrum CBD oil

½ cup (71 g) great quality sauerkraut, drained

1 teaspoon lemon zest

1½ teaspoons Maldon sea salt

METHOD OF PREPARATION:

1. Toast the bread to your desired degree of doneness.

2. While the bread toasts, scoop the avocado flesh into a small bowl, add the desired amount of CBD oil, and mash the ingredients well to combine. Spread half the mashed avocado on each piece of toast.

3. Top the avocado mash with sauerkraut and sprinkle with lemon zest and salt.

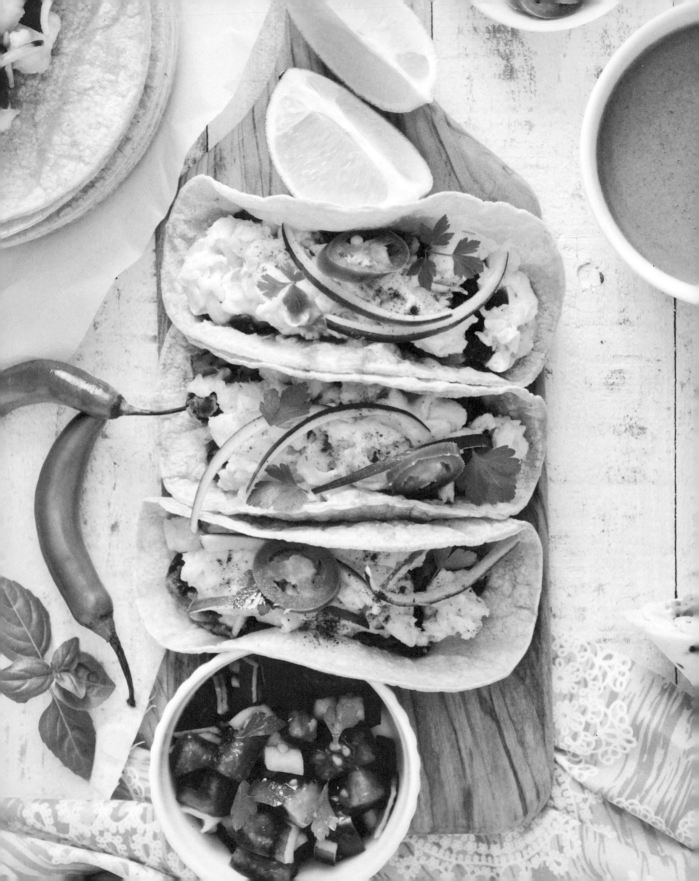

SIMPLE EGG SCRAMBLE
WITH CBD PICO DE GALLO

Yield: Serves 2 / 5 to 10 mg per serving

Simple eggs with bright and tangy Pico de Gallo and a moderate dosage of CBD is a wonderful start to the day. This quick and easy breakfast is great for a chill start to the day.

INGREDIENTS

For Pico de Gallo:
1 cup (180 g) diced tomato
1 tablespoon (10 g) diced red onion
1 tablespoon (10 g) seeded and diced
   jalapeño pepper
1 tablespoon (1 g) fresh cilantro,
   washed and chopped
½ teaspoon sea salt
10 to 20 mg full-spectrum CBD oil

For egg scramble:
4 large eggs, beaten
1 tablespoon (15 ml) water or milk
½ teaspoon sea salt
½ teaspoon freshly ground black
   pepper
1 tablespoon (15 ml) olive oil

TIP *Pico de Gallo is a great addition to so many recipes. Keep this one on hand to spice up tacos, a baked potato, simple quesadillas... honestly it makes everything better!*

METHOD OF PREPARATION:

❶ To make the Pico de Gallo: In a medium bowl, stir together the tomato, red onion, jalapeño, cilantro, salt, and CBD oil. Set aside.

❷ To make the egg scramble: In another medium bowl, whisk the eggs, water, salt, and pepper for 30 to 60 seconds, or until light and fluffy.

❸ Place a medium nonstick sauté pan or skillet over medium-low heat and add the olive oil. Once the pan is warm, add the beaten eggs. Using a rubber spatula, begin pulling the cooked outer edges of the eggs in toward the center of the skillet. Continue this motion until the 3 eggs have reached your desired degree of doneness.

❹ Divide the eggs between two plates and top with the Pico de Gallo.

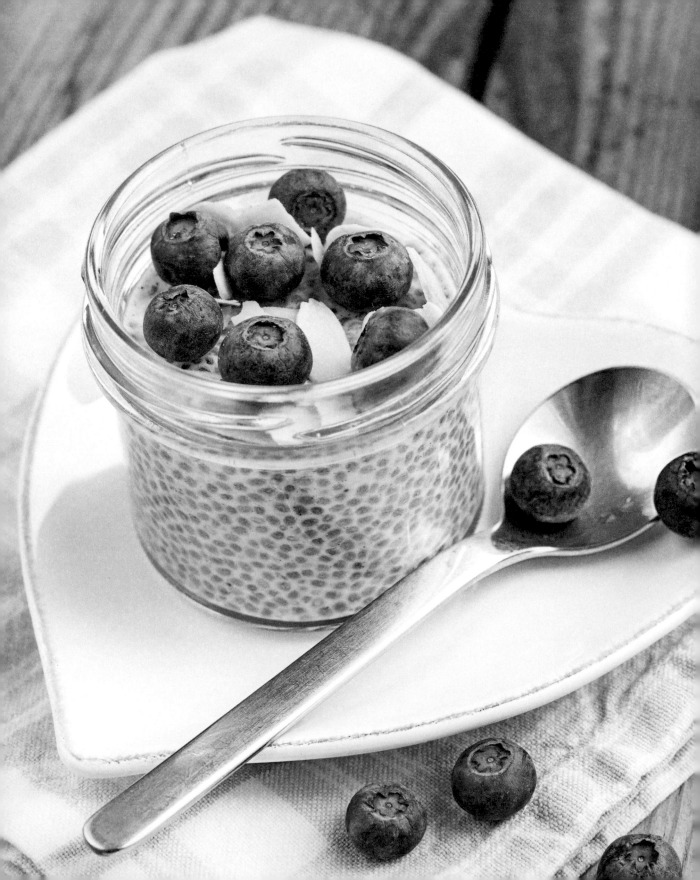

CBD-INFUSED
VANILLA CHIA PUDDING

Yield: Serves 2 / 7 mg per serving

*Who doesn't love chia pudding?!
For breakfast or even for dessert,
this moderate does CBD chia pudding
is the perfect start or end to a day.
Garnish with fruit to really jazz this chia
pudding up.*

INGREDIENTS

2 cups (480 ml) vanilla hemp milk
1 tablespoon (20 g) pure maple syrup
**1 ½ teaspoon (21 g) CBD-infused
    coconut oil**
6 tablespoons (72 g) chia seeds
½ teaspoon vanilla extract
½ teaspoon ground cinnamon
½ teaspoon ground cardamom
¼ teaspoon sea salt

TIP   *Many health food stores now
have CBD infused coconut
oil. If you cannot find it, add 20 mg of
full-spectrum CBD oil to the recipe and
continue with 1½ tablespoons of coconut
oil. The best way to store chia seeds is in
a glass mason jar with a tight-fitting lid
in the refrigerator.*

METHOD OF PREPARATION:

❶   In a medium saucepan over medium heat,
    warm the milk and maple syrup until just
    warmed through. Transfer the mixture to a
    glass jar and stir in the coconut oil and or
    CBD oil.

❷   Add the chia seeds, vanilla, and spices. Cover
    the jar and shake, shake, shake. Refrigerate for
    3 hours, or overnight, before serving.

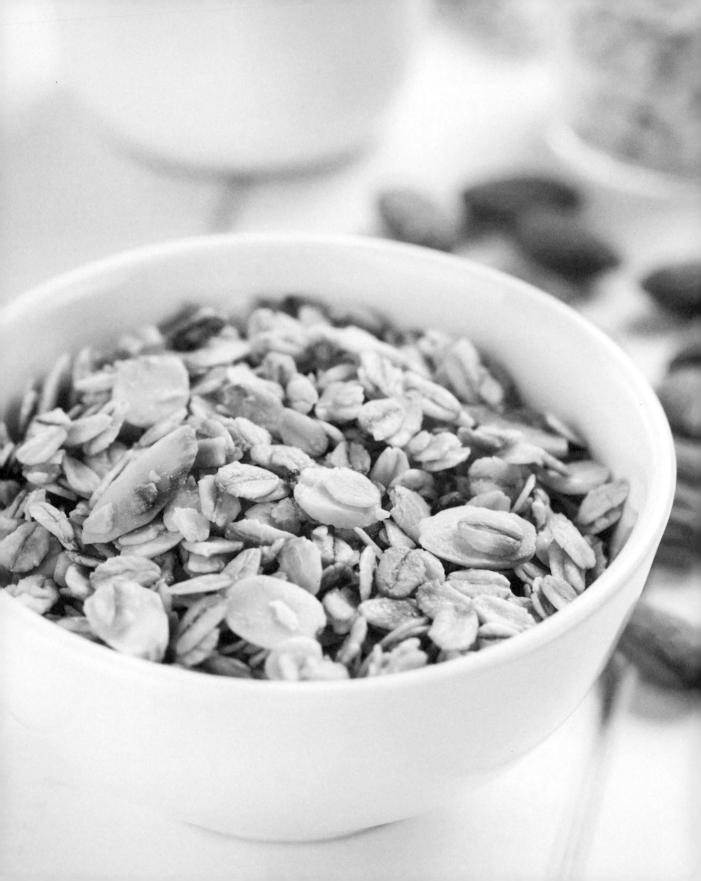

CBD COCONUT-NUT
GRANOLA

Yield: Makes 6 cups, ⅓ cup serving size / about 8 to 11 mg per serving

This granola is a perfect one to make and keep in the freezer for a last-minute nutritious breakfast. The dosage is moderate so try this one to start your day when you are fighting a little inflammation or anxiety.

INGREDIENTS

4 cups (320 g) old-fashioned rolled oats
1 cup (110 g) slivered almonds
1 teaspoon ground cinnamon
1 teaspoon sea salt
¼ teaspoon ground cardamom
½ cup (112 g) coconut oil, melted
½ cup (160 g) coconut nectar or maple syrup
1 teaspoon vanilla extract
½ cup (40 g) unsweetened coconut flakes
½ cup (40 g) unsweetened shredded coconut
150 to 200 mg full-spectrum CBD oil

METHOD OF PREPARATION:

❶ Preheat the oven to 350°F (180°C) and line a large rimmed baking sheet with parchment paper. Set aside.

❷ In a large bowl, stir together the oats, almonds, cinnamon, salt, and cardamom. Add the coconut oil, coconut nectar, and vanilla. Using a rubber spatula, stir until everything is evenly and well coated.

❸ Scrape everything onto the prepared baking sheet and spread it into an even layer. Bake for 15 minutes. Add the coconut flakes and shredded coconut and stir to combine.

❹ Bake for 7 to 10 minutes more, or until the coconut is golden brown.

❺ Let the granola cool completely on the pan.

❻ Once the granola is cool, add the CBD oil and mix thoroughly.

❼ Store the granola in an airtight container. At room temperature, the granola will keep for one to two weeks, or in the freezer for up to three months.

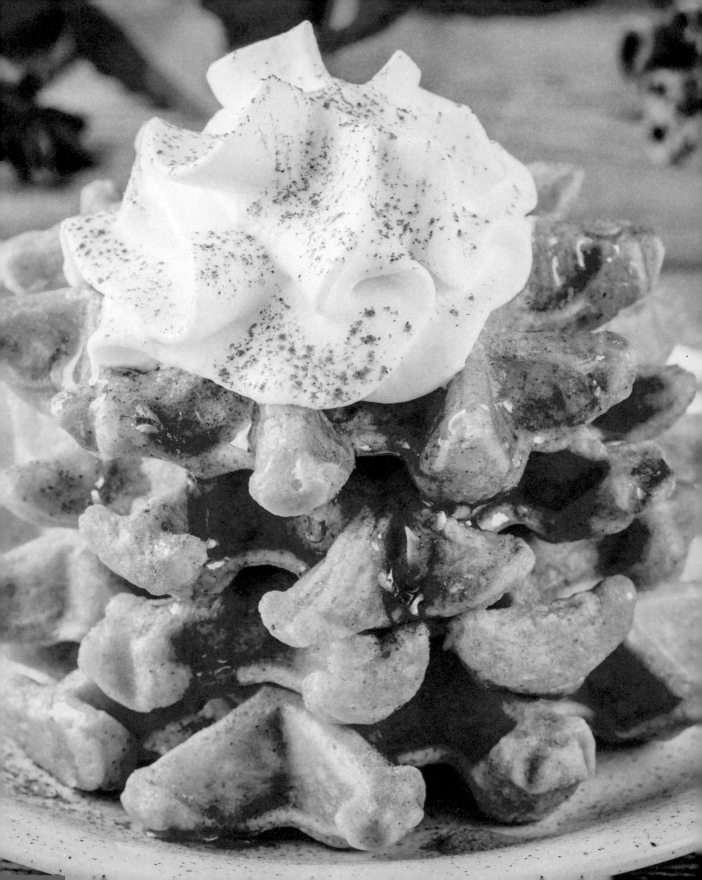

SWEET POTATO HASH BROWN WAFFLES WITH CBD COCONUT WHIPPED CREAM

Yield: Serves 2 / 10 mg CBD per serving

This is a special breakfast, but so worth the effort. The whipped coconut cream is something to use on any and all desserts. This is a moderate CBD dose.

INGREDIENTS

For sweet potato hash brown waffles:
1½ cups (225 g) peeled, grated sweet potato
2 tablespoons (14 g) coconut flour
1 teaspoon sea salt
1 teaspoon ground cinnamon
2 large eggs, beaten, or 6 tablespoons (90 ml) aquafaba*
Nonstick cooking spray, for preparing the waffle iron

For CBD coconut whipped cream:
1 (14 ounces, or 425 ml) can coconut cream, chilled overnight
2 tablespoons (15 g) organic powdered sugar
1 teaspoon vanilla extract
20 mg full-spectrum CBD oil

* *Aquafaba is the liquid from a can of chickpeas and it is an incredible substitute for eggs!*

METHOD OF PREPARATION:

1. Preheat a waffle iron to medium heat.

2. To make the sweet potato hash brown waffles: In a large bowl, stir together the sweet potato, coconut flour, salt, cinnamon, and eggs until thoroughly combined.

3. Spray the waffle iron with cooking spray. Spoon the batter into the center of the iron and spread it outward. Close the iron and cook for 6 to 8 minutes, or until the waffle is browned and crispy.

4. Remove the waffle, keep warm, and repeat with the remaining batter.

5. To make the CBD coconut whipped cream: While the waffles cook, place the chilled coconut cream and powdered sugar in a large bowl or in the bowl of a stand mixer fitted with the balloon whisk attachment. Whisk on high speed with a handheld electric mixer or the stand mixer for 1 minute, or until fluffy.

6. Add the vanilla and CBD oil and continue whisking for 30 seconds more, or until the CBD oil is fully dispersed. Cover and chill until ready to serve.

7. Top the warm waffles with the coconut cream.

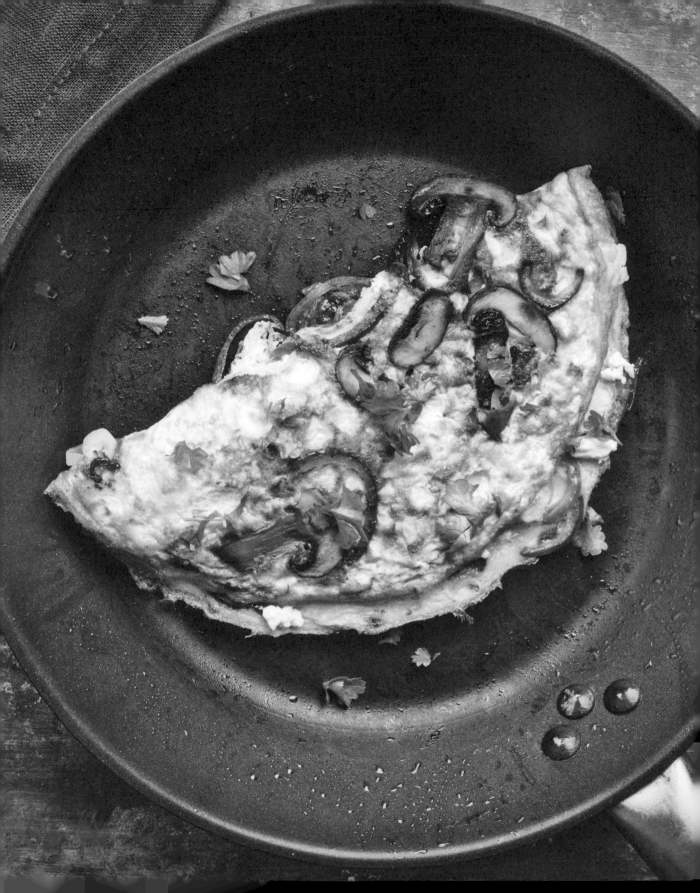

ULTIMATE FRENCH OMELET
WITH ROASTED MUSHROOMS, HERBS & CBD OIL

Yield: Serves 1 / 10 mg per serving

Oh, the perfect omelet. This method is based upon Julia Child's method and it makes the lightest fluffiest omelet, shaking the pan is the secret. This is a moderate dose of CBD.

INGREDIENTS

3 large eggs
1 teaspoon cold water
1 teaspoon sea salt
½ teaspoon freshly ground black
    pepper
1 tablespoon (14 g) unsalted butter
½ cup (84 g) roasted wild mushrooms
1 tablespoon (4 g) chopped fresh Italian
    parsley
1 tablespoon (2.5 g) chopped fresh basil
10 mg full-spectrum CBD oil

METHOD OF PREPARATION:

1. In a medium bowl, whisk the eggs, water, salt, and pepper and set aside.

2. Place a medium nonstick skillet over high heat. Add the butter to melt, tilting the pan in all directions to coat the bottom and sides. When the foam has almost subsided, but before the butter browns, pour in the eggs.

3. Tilt and shake the pan briefly to spread the eggs over the bottom of the pan, then let the pan sit for a few seconds without shaking it while the eggs cook and begin to firm on the bottom. Place the mushrooms, herbs, and CBD oil in the center of the omelet.

4. Start jerking the pan toward you, making the eggs hit the far edge of the pan. Continue this motion as the omelet begins to roll over itself. Use a rubber spatula to push up any egg, as needed. Then bang the pan so the omelet starts curling over the edge.

5. Fold the omelet into thirds and transfer it to a plate to serve.

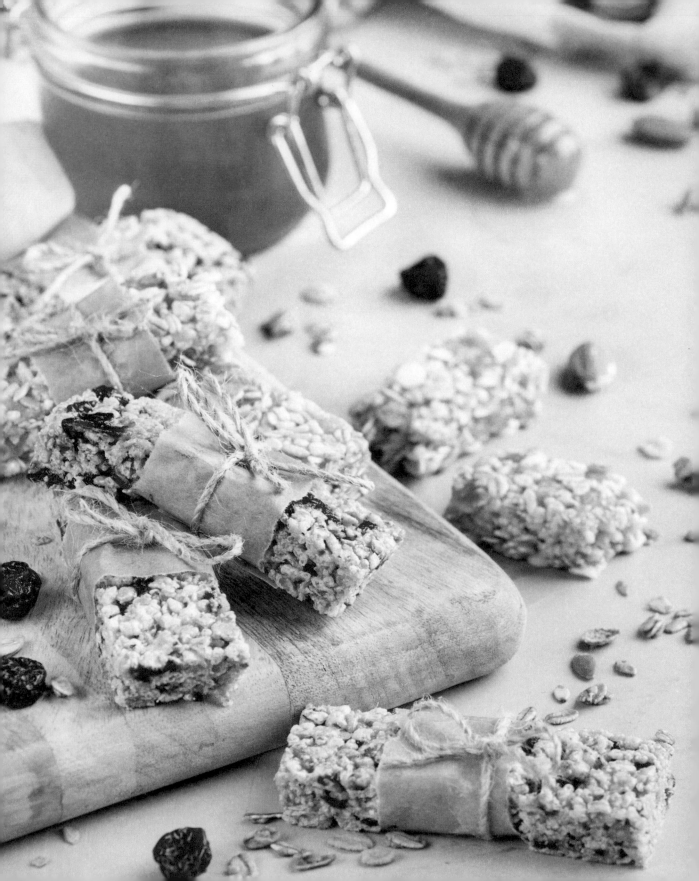

NO-BAKE OATS & HONEY
CBD BREAKFAST BARS

Yield: Serves 8 / 6 to 12 mg per serving

These no bake breakfast bars are so simple to make and a delicious grab and go breakfast or snack. They are low to moderate on the CBD dosage and make a perfect calming start to your day.

INGREDIENTS

½ cup (160 g) honey
50 to 100 mg full-spectrum CBD oil
¼ cup (65 g) almond butter
3 cups (84 g) toasted oat cereal
½ cup (72.5 g) unsalted almonds,
    toasted and chopped
½ cup (60 g) dried cranberries

TIP *Make these no bake bars with peanut butter, cashew butter, or sunflower seed butter to switch things up!*

METHOD OF PREPARATION:

❶ Line an 8 x 8-inch (20 x 20 cm) baking pan with parchment paper and set aside. In a medium microwave-safe bowl, stir together the honey, CBD oil, and almond butter.

❷ Microwave the mixture on high power for 45 seconds, stirring every 15 seconds, or until melted.

❸ In a large bowl, combine the cereal, almonds, and cranberries. Pour the melted honey mixture over the cereal mixture and stir until well mixed. Pour the batter into the prepared pan, pressing it in evenly.

❹ Transfer the pan to the freezer for about 30 minutes.

❺ Once the mixture is hard, cut it into eight pieces. Wrap each bar in parchment paper and keep refrigerated for 1 week or freeze for up to three months.

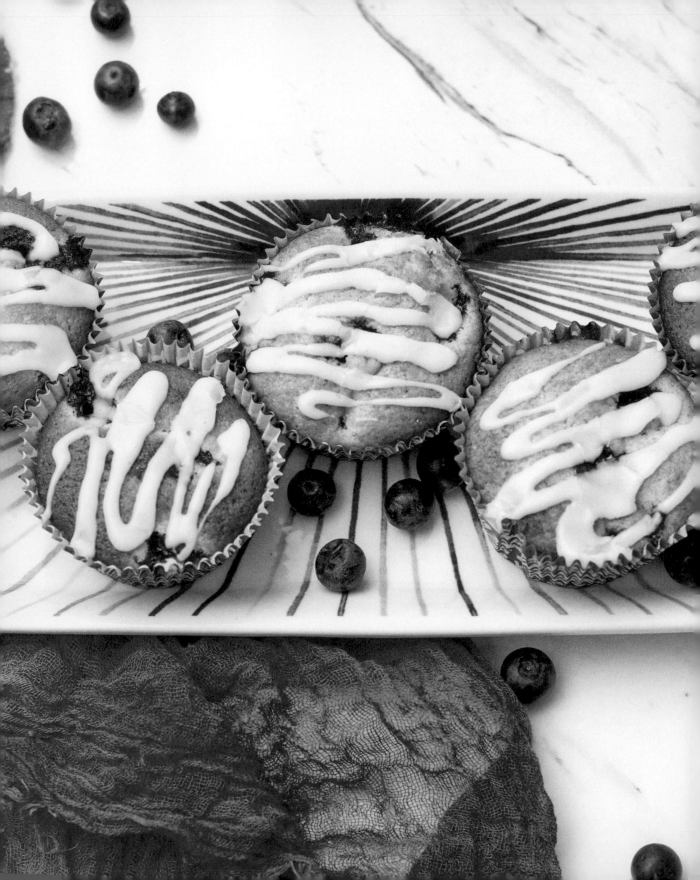

CBD GLAZED
BLUEBERRY MUFFINS

Yield: Serves 12 / 8 to 12.5 mg per muffin

These muffins, whether you choose to make them vegan or not, are a perfect grab and go breakfast for a calm, anxiety free day.

INGREDIENTS

For the muffins:
½ cup (112 g) coconut oil, melted
4 cups (496 g) all-purpose flour
1½ cups (300 g) organic sugar
2 tablespoons (27.5 g) baking powder
1 teaspoon kosher salt
2 large eggs or 6 tablespoons (90 ml) aquafaba*
2 cups (480 ml) hemp milk
2 cups (290 g) fresh blueberries, washed and dried
1 tablespoon (6 g) orange zest

For the CBD glaze:
I cup confectioner's sugar
I tablespoon pure vanilla extract
100 to 150 mg full-spectrum CBD oil
½ cup unsweetened almond milk

* Aquafaba is the liquid from a can of chickpeas and it is an incredible substitute for eggs!

METHOD OF PREPARATION:

❶ Preheat the oven to 400°F. Line a muffin pan with liners and set aside.

❷ In a large bowl, whisk the flour, sugar, baking powder, and salt. In a medium bowl, whisk the eggs, milk, and coconut oil.

❸ Stir the wet ingredients into the dry ingredients just until incorporated; do not overmix. The batter will be lumpy. Fold in the blueberries and orange zest. Spoon the batter into the prepared muffin pan.

❹ Bake for 25 minutes, or until a toothpick inserted into a muffin comes out clean and the muffins are lightly golden brown.

❺ To make the glaze: in a medium bowl, combine the confectioner's sugar, vanilla, and CBD oil. Slowly whisk in the almond milk.

❻ Cool on a wire rack, brush with the glaze, and enjoy.

CARROT CAKE
BREAKFAST BREAD WITH CBD GLAZE

Yield: Serves 12 / about 8 to 17 mg per serving

This hearty breakfast bread with a CBD glaze is the ultimate weekend treat. Whether you had a late night out, a major weekend workout, or just need a calm Sunday brunch, this is for you. Start on the lower end of the CBD spectrum and work your way up!

INGREDIENTS

For the carrot cake:
1½ cups (144 g) whole-wheat pastry flour
½ cup (40 g) quick oats
2 teaspoons ground cinnamon
1 teaspoon baking powder
¾ teaspoon baking soda
½ teaspoon freshly grated nutmeg
½ teaspoon sea salt
2 medium bananas, mashed
½ cup (72 g) coconut sugar
1 large egg
1 teaspoon vanilla extract
¼ cup (60 g) unsweetened applesauce
⅓ cup (80 ml) vanilla almond milk or hemp milk
1 cup (110 g) shredded carrot
2 tablespoons (28 g) coconut oil, melted and cooled slightly
¼ cup (25 g) walnuts, chopped
¼ cup (37 g) raisins

For the CBD glaze:
4 ounces (115 g) almond yogurt or cashew yogurt
⅓ cup (40 g) organic powdered sugar
¼ teaspoon ground cinnamon
½ teaspoon vanilla extract
100 to 200 mg full-spectrum CBD oil

METHOD OF PREPARATION:

❶ To make the carrot cake: Preheat the oven to 350°F (180°C). Spray a 9 x 5-inch (23 x 13 cm) loaf pan with nonstick cooking spray and set aside.

❷ In a large bowl, whisk the flour, oats, cinnamon, baking powder, baking soda, nutmeg, and salt. Set aside.

❸ In a medium bowl, stir together the mashed banana, coconut sugar, egg, and vanilla until well combined and creamy.

❹ Stir in the applesauce and milk and fold in the carrot. Add the wet ingredients to the dry ingredients and mix until just combined. Do not overmix.

❺ Gently fold in the coconut oil, walnuts, and raisins.

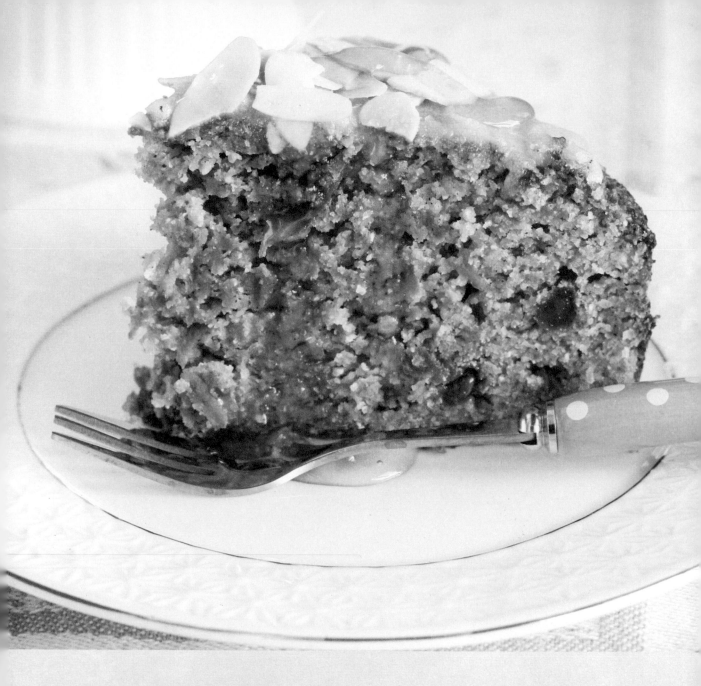

6 Pour the batter into the prepared loaf pan and bake for 45 to 60 minutes, or until a toothpick inserted into the center comes out clean with a few crumbs attached. Transfer to a wire rack to cool for 15 minutes. Remove the loaf from the pan and place on the wire rack to finish cooling completely.

7 To make the glaze: In a medium bowl, combine all the glaze ingredients and whisk to combine. Spread over the cooled bread and slice the loaf into 12 pieces.

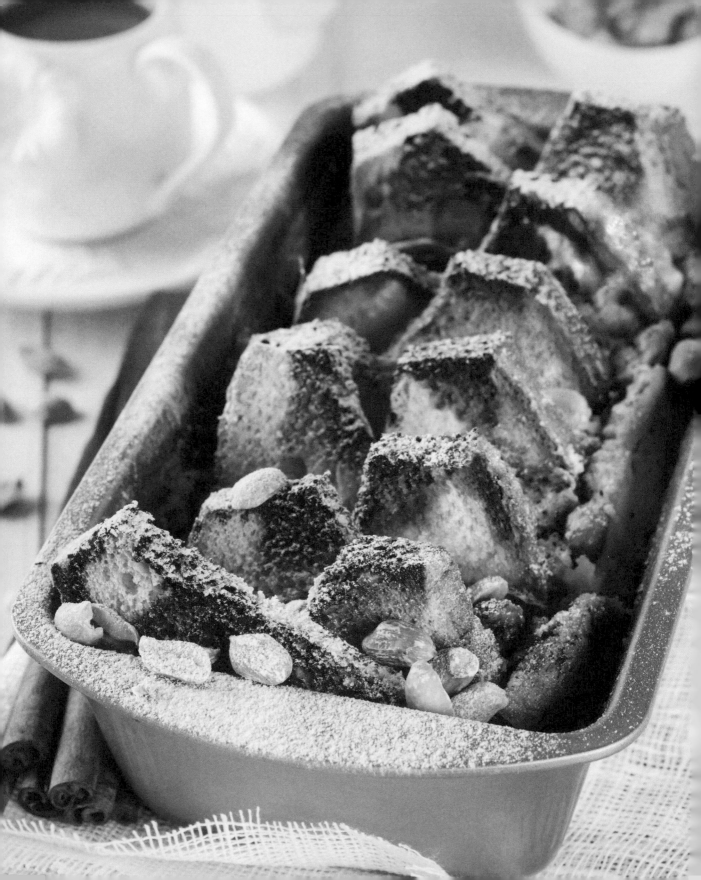

RECOVERY CBD-INFUSED
FRENCH TOAST CASSEROLE

Yield: Serves 12 / about 33 to 50 mg CBD per serving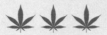

This breakfast is perfect for a recovery day. Whether you are an athlete or had an extreme workout, the amount of CBD in this casserole will help with inflammation and allow the muscles to recover quickly.

INGREDIENTS

Nonstick cooking spray, for preparing the baking dish
1 brioche loaf, cut into 1-inch (2.5 cm) cubes
1 (12 ounces, or 340 g) container mascarpone or dairy-free cream cheese, such as Kite Hill
2 cups (480 ml) hemp milk
1 cup (240 ml) heavy cream or plant-based half-and-half
8 large eggs
2 tablespoons (25 g) organic sugar
1 teaspoon vanilla extract
½ teaspoon ground cinnamon
¼ teaspoon freshly grated nutmeg
⅛ teaspoon salt
400 to 600 mg full-spectrum CBD oil

TIP *Make this casserole the night before and bake in the morning for a super simple and elegant breakfast.*

METHOD OF PREPARATION:

❶ Coat a 9 x 13-inch (23 x 33 cm) baking dish with cooking spray.

❷ Arrange two-thirds of the bread cubes in the prepared baking dish and dot evenly with the mascarpone. Top with the remaining bread cubes and press down gently. In a large bowl, whisk the milk, heavy cream, eggs, sugar, vanilla, cinnamon, nutmeg, salt, and CBD oil.

❸ Pour the mixture evenly over the casserole. Cover and refrigerate for 3 hours, or overnight.

❹ When ready to bake, preheat the oven to 350°F (180°C).

❺ Uncover the casserole and bake for 40 to 50 minutes, or until lightly browned and puffy.

❻ Let rest for 10 minutes before serving.

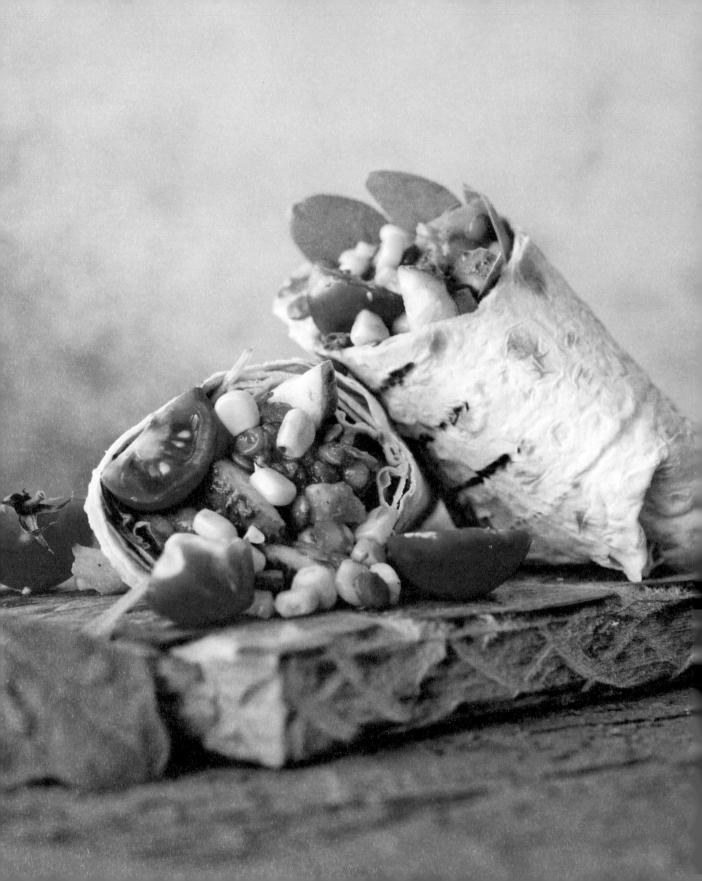

CBD-INFUSED
VEGGIE BREAKFAST BURRITO

Yield: Serves 4 / 20 to 50 mg per serving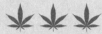

This high-dose breakfast burrito is perfect pre-workout to stop sore muscles and inflammation in their tracks or post-workout for a smooth sailing recovery. Either way, it's packed full of delicious nutrient-dense vegetables for a wonderful and filling breakfast.

INGREDIENTS

2 tablespoons (30 ml) avocado oil
1 sweet onion, diced
1 cup (96 g) cremini mushrooms, cleaned and sliced
2 cups (220 g) peeled, diced Japanese yam
1 cup (240 ml) water
1 teaspoon ground cumin
1 teaspoon chili powder
1 teaspoon sea salt
½ teaspoon freshly ground black pepper
1 (1 pound, or 454 g) container silken tofu, drained and crumbled
4 cups (120 g) fresh baby spinach leaves
1 cup (260 g) prepared salsa, plus more for serving
80 to 200 mg full-spectrum CBD oil
4 burrito-size tortillas
½ cup (60 g) shredded cheddar cheese or dairy-free cheese
4 avocados, peeled, pitted, and sliced

METHOD OF PREPARATION:

❶ Heat a large nonstick sauté pan or skillet over medium-high heat. Add the avocado oil, onion, mushrooms, yam, water, cumin, chili powder, salt, and pepper. Sauté for 15 to 20 minutes, or until the water evaporates and the vegetables are tender.

❷ Add the tofu, spinach, and salsa. Cook, stirring, for 3 minutes, or until the spinach wilts.

❸ Turn off the heat and stir in the CBD oil.

❹ Place the tortillas on a work surface and evenly divide the mixture among them. Sprinkle with the shredded cheddar cheese. Fold the two ends in and then the sides over and wrap tightly to form a burrito. Heat a griddle over medium heat. Place the burritos, folded-side down, in the pan and cook until crispy, 4 to 5 minutes. Flip and cook for 4 to 5 minutes more on the other side.

❺ Serve hot with extra salsa and avocado.

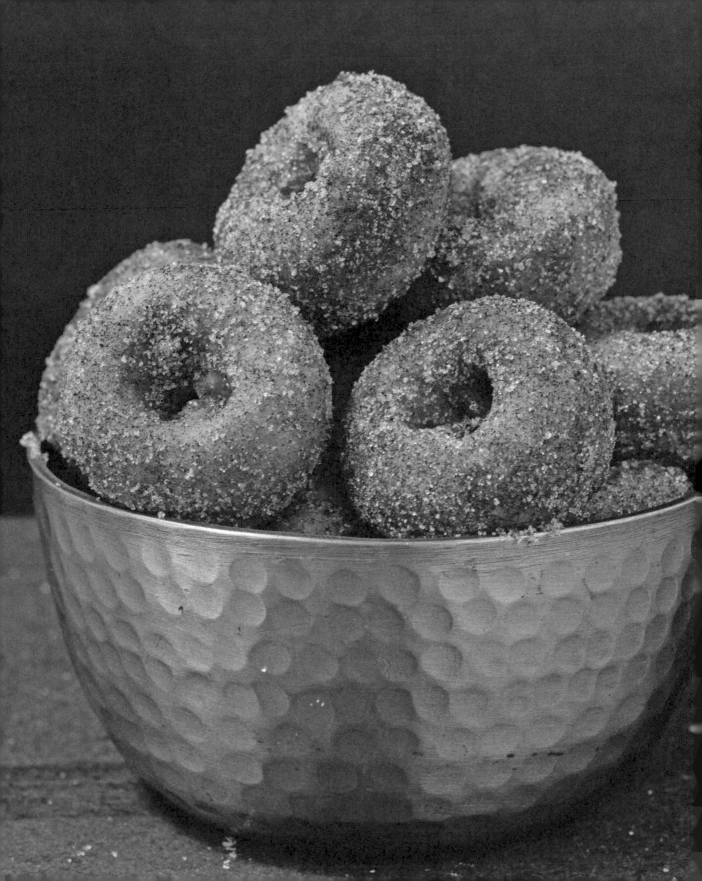

CINNAMON BAKED
DOUGHNUTS WITH CBD SUGAR COATING

Yield: Serves 12 / 25 to 42 mg CBD per serving

Doughnuts! These baked doughnuts are a special treat. They are on the high side of CBD, so lower the amount of oil if you wish to have a more chill baked good experience.

INGREDIENTS

For the doughnuts:
Nonstick baking spray
2 cups (248 g) all-purpose flour
1½ cups (300 g) organic sugar
2 teaspoons baking powder
1 teaspoon ground cinnamon
½ teaspoon sea salt
1 extra-large egg, beaten
1¼ cups (300 ml) vanilla hemp milk
2 tablespoons (28 g) unsalted butter or
  dairy-free butter, melted
2 teaspoons vanilla extract

For the CBD sugar coating:
8 tablespoons (112 g) unsalted butter or
  dairy-free butter
300 to 500 mg full-spectrum CBD oil
½ cup (100 g) organic sugar
1 teaspoon ground cinnamon

METHOD OF PREPARATION:

❶ Preheat the oven to 350°F (180°C). Generously coat two doughnut pans with baking spray and set aside.

❷ In a large bowl, sift together the flour, sugar, baking powder, cinnamon, and salt. In a medium bowl, whisk the egg, milk, melted butter, and vanilla. Add the wet ingredients to the dry ingredients and stir with a wooden spoon until just combined.

❸ Spoon the batter into the prepared pans, filling each one a little more than three-quarters full.

❹ Bake for 15 to 17 minutes, or until a toothpick inserted into the doughnuts comes out clean.

❺ Let cool for 5 minutes. Invert the pans onto a sheet pan and tap the doughnuts out onto it.

❻ To make the CBD sugar coating: In a medium sauté pan or skillet over medium-low heat, melt the butter.

❼ Remove from the heat and whisk in the CBD.

❽ In a small bowl, stir together the sugar and cinnamon.

❾ To finish the doughnuts, dip them in the CBD butter and then into the cinnamon sugar, coating both sides.

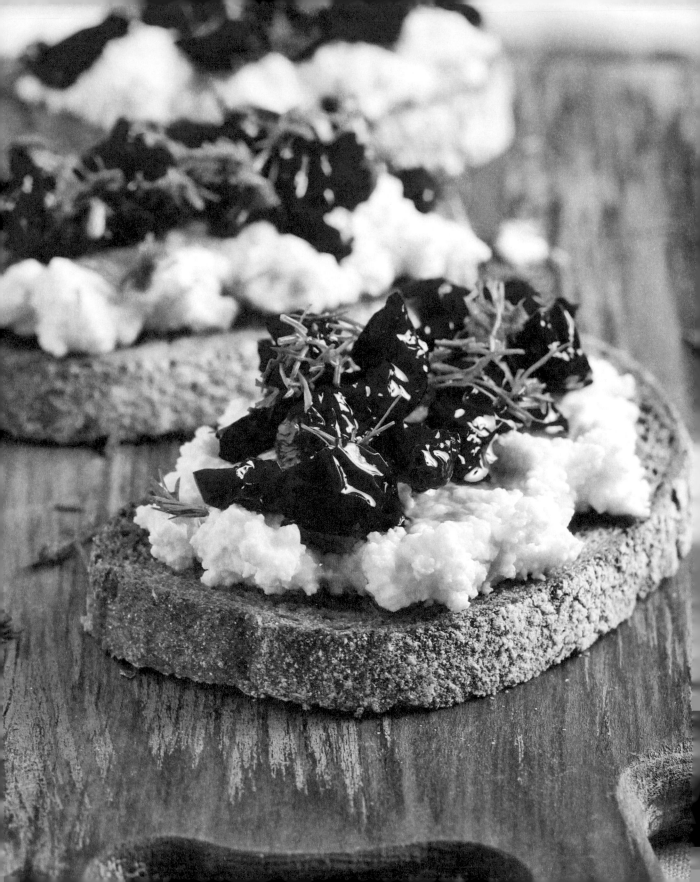

TOMATO TOAST WITH MACADAMIA, RICOTTA & CBD-INFUSED HONEY DRIZZLE

Yield: Serves 12 / about 17 to 33 mg per serving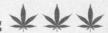

What an incredible and special brunch! This one takes some time to prepare, but you will love the combination of creamy, crunchy, sweet and savory. This is a high CBD dose and should be used for inflammation recovery or to soothe super sore muscles.

INGREDIENTS

For the macadamia ricotta:
2 cups (270 g) raw macadamia nuts
1 teaspoon kosher salt
1 tablespoon (15 ml) fresh lemon juice
½ cup (120 ml) water, plus more as
    needed

For the tomato toast:
2 plum tomatoes, seeded and diced
3 tablespoons (45 ml) olive oil
2 tablespoons (8 g) fresh parsley,
    chopped
¼ teaspoon freshly ground black pepper
¼ teaspoon sea salt
1 (8 ounces, or 225 g) loaf Italian bread,
    sliced diagonally into ½-inch (1 cm)-
    thick slices

For the CBD-infused honey:
½ cup (160 g) raw local honey
200 to 400 mg full-spectrum CBD oil

METHOD OF PREPARATION:

❶ To make the macadamia ricotta: In a food processor or a high-powered blender, combine all the ricotta ingredients and purée until smooth, stopping to scrape down the sides and add a bit more water, if needed. The texture should resemble dairy ricotta. Set aside.

❷ To make the tomato toast: Preheat the oven to 400°F (200°C). Line a sheet pan with parchment paper and set aside.

❸ In a medium bowl, stir together the tomatoes, olive oil, parsley, pepper, and salt.

❹ Place the bread slices on the prepared baking sheet and bake for 5 minutes, or until golden brown.

❺ To make the CBD-infused honey: While the bread toasts, in a small microwavable bowl, microwave the honey on high power for 20 to 30 seconds. Let cool slightly and whisk in the CBD oil. Set aside.

❻ When ready to serve, top the toasted bread with some of the tomato mixture followed by a dollop of the macadamia ricotta and drizzle with the honey.

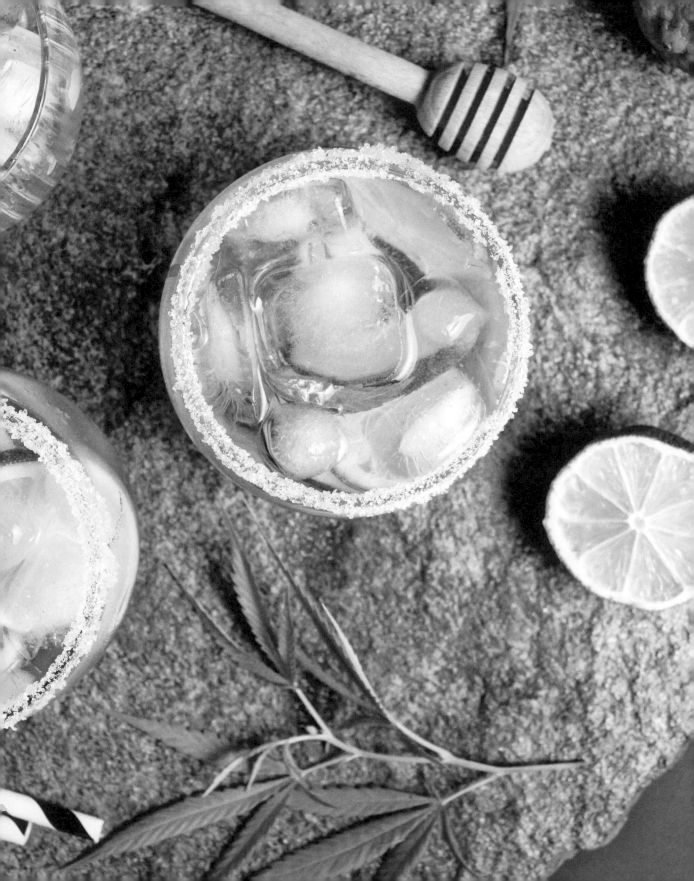

DRINKS

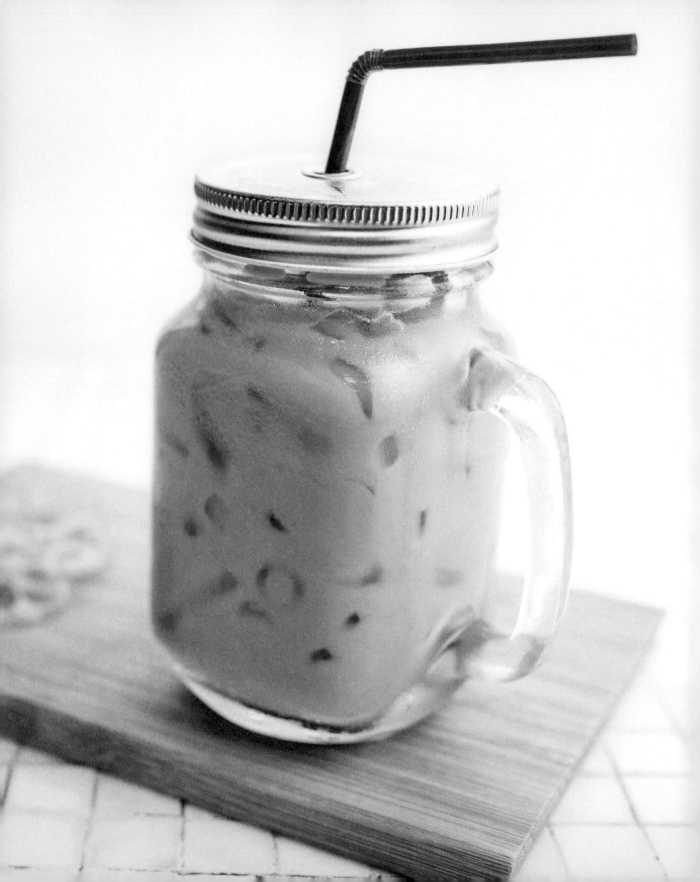

CBD-INFUSED
RUM THAI ICED TEA

Yield: Serves 4 / 5 mg CBD per serving

Thai Iced Tea is so delicious on its own, but add in some rum and CBD and you have a relaxing cocktail on a whole new level. This is a low CBD dosage beverage.

INGREDIENTS

4 cups (960 ml) filtered water
2 tablespoons (4 g) loose leaf black tea leaves
¼ cup (80 g) coconut nectar
¼ cup (60 g) packed organic light brown sugar
20 mg full-spectrum or water-soluble CBD oil
1 teaspoon vanilla extract
½ cup (120 ml) dark rum
1 (14 ounces, or 425 ml) can coconut milk

TIP *If you can't find coconut nectar or don't have it on hand, you may substitute maple syrup or brown rice syrup.*

METHOD OF PREPARATION:

❶ In a large saucepan over high heat, bring the water to a boil. Once boiling, remove from the heat. Stir in the tea and let steep for 5 minutes.

❷ Set a fine-mesh strainer over a pitcher and pour the tea through it to remove the loose tea leaves. Discard the leaves. Stir in the coconut nectar, brown sugar, and CBD oil, stirring until the sugar dissolves and the CBD oil is incorporated.

❸ Transfer the tea to the refrigerator and chill for 2 to 3 hours.

❹ Stir in the vanilla.

❺ To serve, fill four glasses with ice and divide the chilled tea among the glasses. Pour 2 tablespoons of rum on top of the tea in each glass. Divide the coconut milk among the glasses and let guests stir it in themselves.

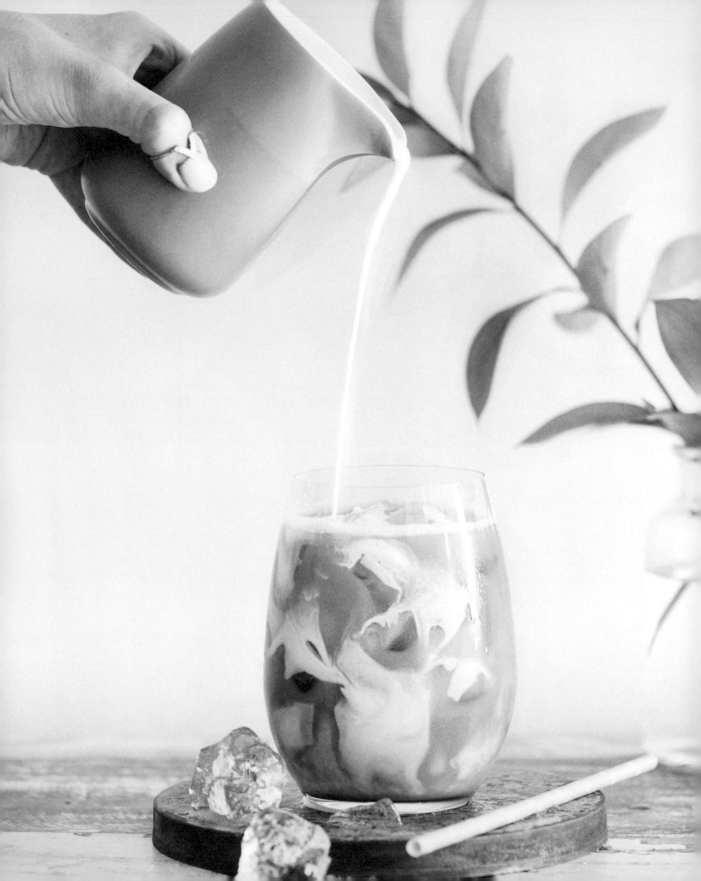

COCONUT MATCHA
CBD TEA LATTE

Yield: Serves 2 / 5 to 10 mg CBD per serving

This is by far one of my favorite lattes! The sweetness of the coconut, the complexity of the matcha, the creaminess of the macadamia milk, the low dosage of CBD...this is a perfect start to the day.

INGREDIENTS

2 teaspoons organic ceremonial-grade
    matcha powder
10 to 20 mg full-spectrum CBD oil
2 tablespoons (40 g) maple syrup
1 cup (240 ml) macadamia milk
2 cups (480 ml) hot water, not boiling
2 teaspoons virgin coconut oil (optional)

TIP   *Make sure you buy ceremonial-grade Matcha. It is expensive, but well worth the investment.*

METHOD OF PREPARATION:

1. In a blender, combine all the ingredients, including the coconut oil (if using), and blend on high speed for 15 to 20 seconds, or until well combined and frothy.

2. Serve hot or chill and serve over ice.

FRUITY PARTY VODKA
CBD PUNCH

Yield: Serves 16 / about 5 mg CBD per serving

Having a party? Want to make an extra special signature drink? This is the one for you! An easy fruit punch with a low CBD dose.

INGREDIENTS

6 ounces (170 g) frozen lemonade concentrate, thawed
6 ounces (170 g) frozen fruit punch concentrate, thawed
½ cup (80 g) drained red Maraschino cherries
1 cup (165 g) fresh pineapple chunks
1 quart (960 ml) club soda
1 cup (240 ml) vodka
½ cup (120 ml) light rum
75 to 80 mg full-spectrum or water-soluble CBD oil

METHOD OF PREPARATION:

❶ In a large pitcher, combine all the ingredients and stir to mix.

❷ Serve over ice.

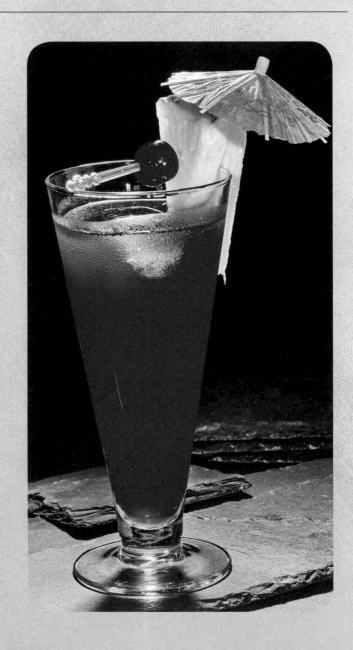

MINT & WATERMELON
CBD MOJITO

Yield: Serves 2 / 10 mg CBD per serving

This is one of my favorite summer cocktails. Make this when watermelon is at its peak and get ready to enjoy a hydrating, delicious and relaxing cocktail. This beverage is a moderate CBD dose.

INGREDIENTS

8 fresh mint leaves, loosely torn
1 tablespoon (20 g) raw local honey
20 mg full-spectrum or water-soluble CBD oil
2 tablespoons (30 ml) fresh lime juice
½ cup (120 ml) light rum
1 cup (240 ml) fresh watermelon juice
1 cup (240 ml) soda water

METHOD OF PREPARATION:

❶   In a mortar and pestle, mash together the mint leaves, honey, and CBD oil. Add the lime juice and stir to combine.

❷   Divide the mint mixture between two glasses and top with ice.

❸   Pour ¼ cup (60 ml) of rum into each glass. Top each with ½ cup (120 ml) of watermelon juice and ½ cup (120 ml) of soda water. Stir and serve.

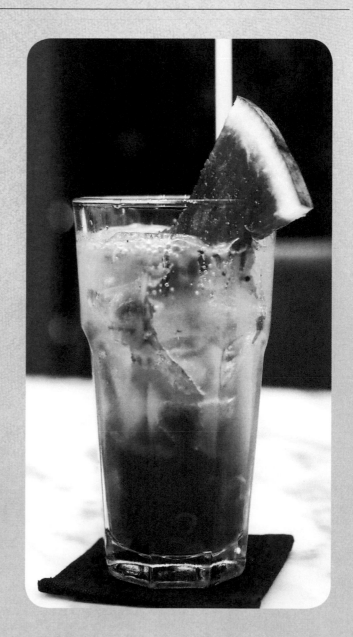

CBD GINGER-TURMERIC
GOLDEN MILK

Yield: Serves 2 / 10 mg CBD per serving

This is one of the most nourishing drinks, it's a natural anti-inflammatory, hydrating, antibacterial, antimicrobial, and relaxing. This is a low CBD dose.

INGREDIENTS

1 tablespoon (8 g) fresh turmeric root, peeled and grated
1 tablespoon (8 g) fresh ginger, peeled and grated
2 teaspoons ghee
10 to 20 mg full-spectrum CBD oil
1 cup (240 ml) full-fat coconut milk
1 cup (240 ml) coconut water
1 tablespoon (20 g) Manuka honey

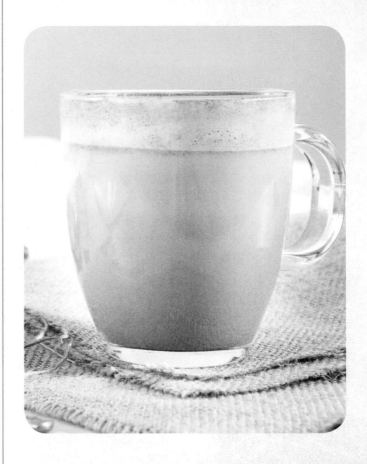

METHOD OF PREPARATION:

❶ In a small bowl, combine the turmeric, ginger, ghee, and CBD oil. Using a fork, mix together well, mashing to form a fine paste.

❷ In a medium saucepan over medium heat, combine the coconut milk, coconut water, and spice paste. Cook, whisking, until heated. Do not boil. Once tiny bubbles begin to appear on the side of the pan, turn off the heat, cover the pan, and let the tea steep for 3 minutes.

❸ Stir in the honey and serve.

MOCHA OAT
CBD LATTE

Yield: Serves 2 / 10 mg CBD per serving

Oat milk lattes are all the rage right now. Its super creamy consistency lends perfectly to a relaxing, filling morning beverage. This is moderate CBD dose.

INGREDIENTS

2 cups (480 ml) hot brewed coffee
½ cup (120 ml) warm chocolate oat milk
    or almond milk
2 pitted dates
2 tablespoons (10 g) dark cocoa powder
1 tablespoon (14 g) virgin coconut oil
20 mg full-spectrum CBD oil

METHOD OF PREPARATION:

In a high-powered blender, combine all the ingredients and blend until frothy.

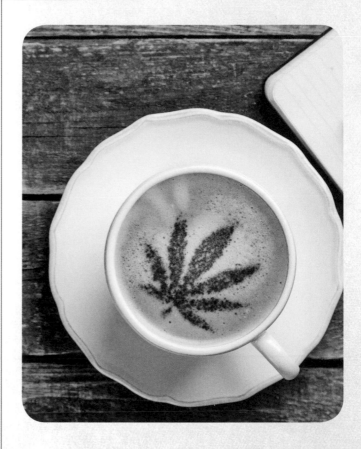

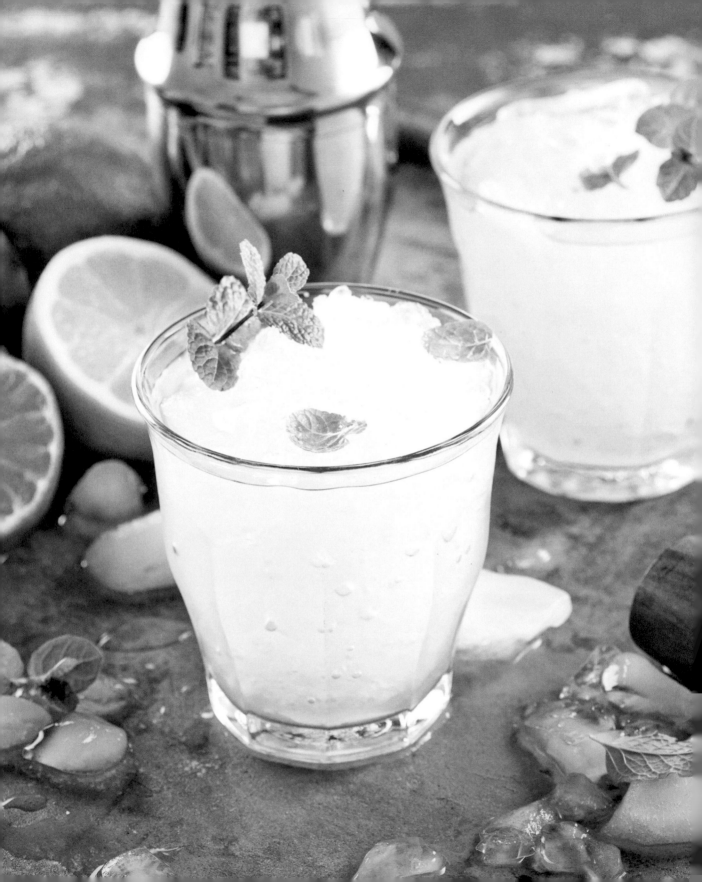

THE UPDATED
MARGARITA

Yield: Serves 4 / 7.5 to 12.5 mg CBD per serving

This margarita is so fresh and delightful. It has a moderate CBD dosage, so drink slowly and enjoy the relaxing benefits.

INGREDIENTS

6 ounces (180 ml) tequila of choice
6 ounces (180 ml) triple sec
4 ounces (120 ml) fresh lime juice
2 ounces (60 ml) fresh orange juice
30 to 50 mg full-spectrum CBD oil
Margarita salt, for rimming the glasses
Orange wedges, for rimming the glasses
Ice, for serving
Lime wedges, for serving

TIP *You can easily double or triple this recipe for a fiesta! Just have your guests help you with the fresh squeezed juice, that's what makes this margarita special.*

METHOD OF PREPARATION:

❶ In a pitcher, combine the tequila, triple sec, lime juice, orange juice, and CBD oil. Stir well to mix.

❷ Place the salt in a shallow dish or plate.

❸ To serve, run an orange wedge around the rim of a glass and dip it into the salt. Shake off any excess. Add ice to the glass and pour the margarita mixture over the ice.

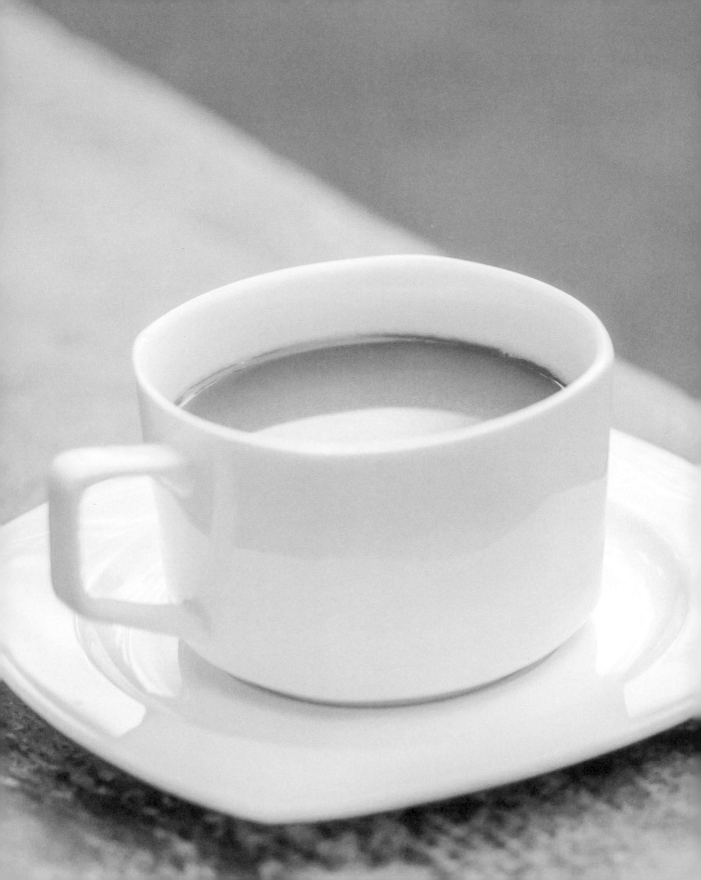

CBD PERIOD RELIEF
TEA LATTE

Yield: Serves 4 / 7.5 to 12.5 mg CBD per serving

CBD is ideal for period relief. This is a moderate CBD dose. This blend of herbs is especially potent for period relief. You can make a large jar and keep this mixture in a cool dry place for an easy PMS/period symptom relief tea.

INGREDIENTS

1 cup (112 g) dandelion root
1 cup (237 g) burdock root
½ cup (50 g) cranberry tea
¼ cup (25 g) sliced fresh ginger, peeled and sliced
2 cups (480 ml) unsweetened milk or hemp milk
2 tablespoons (40 g) maple syrup or coconut nectar
20 to 40 mg full-spectrum CBD oil
⅛ teaspoon ground ginger
⅛ teaspoon ground nutmeg

METHOD OF PREPARATION:

1. In a large glass jar with a lid, such as a Mason jar, combine the dandelion, burdock, cranberry, and fresh ginger.

2. In a medium heavy-bottomed saucepan over medium heat, combine the almond milk and 2 teaspoons of the tea mixture. Heat until hot but not boiling. Strain the milk into a pitcher.

3. Whisk in the maple syrup, coconut nectar, CBD oil, ground ginger, and nutmeg.

4. If you like, using a milk frother, froth until the desired amount of foam is achieved.

5. Store the remaining tea mixture in the sealed jar in a cool, dark place for 6-12 months.

CALMING BERRY VANILLA
CBD SMOOTHIE

Yield: Serves 2 / 10 to 20 mg CBD per serving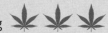

I love a smoothie for dessert. This one is just a simple way to drift off into a peaceful calming sleep, with a high dosage of CBD.

INGREDIENTS

1 cup (250 g) organic frozen raspberries
1 cup (150 g) organic frozen strawberries
½ cup (77.5 g) organic frozen blueberries
2 scoops (20 g) vanilla pea protein
    powder
20 to 40 mg full-spectrum CBD oil
2 cups (480 ml) vanilla hemp milk

METHOD OF PREPARATION:

In a high-powered blender, combine all ingredients in the order listed. Blend on high speed for 30 seconds, or until smooth and creamy.

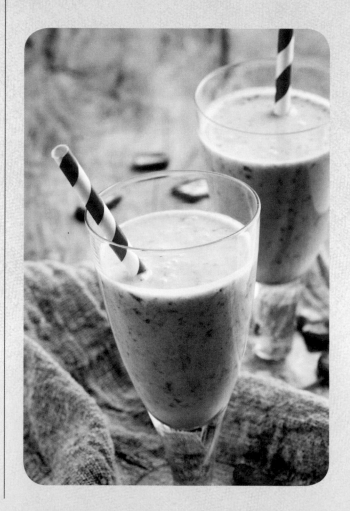

GREEN RECOVERY
CBD SMOOTHIE

Yield: Serves 2 / 25 to 100 mg CBD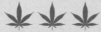

This smoothie is for those post workout recovery needs. Calorie-dense, it is chock full of antioxidants and inflammation-fighting goodness. This is a high CBD dose.

INGREDIENTS

2 cups (280 g) organic frozen pineapple chunks

2 cups (134 g) fresh organic kale

2 cups (60 g) fresh organic baby spinach leaves

½ avocado, peeled and pitted

2 tablespoons (14 g) hemp hearts

50 to 200 mg full-spectrum CBD oil

2½ cups (600 ml) coconut water

METHOD OF PREPARATION:

In a high-powered blender, combine all the ingredients in the order listed. Purée until smooth and creamy.

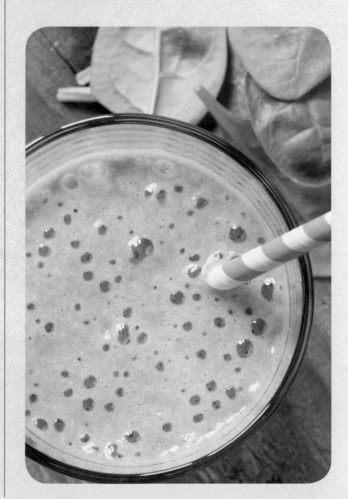

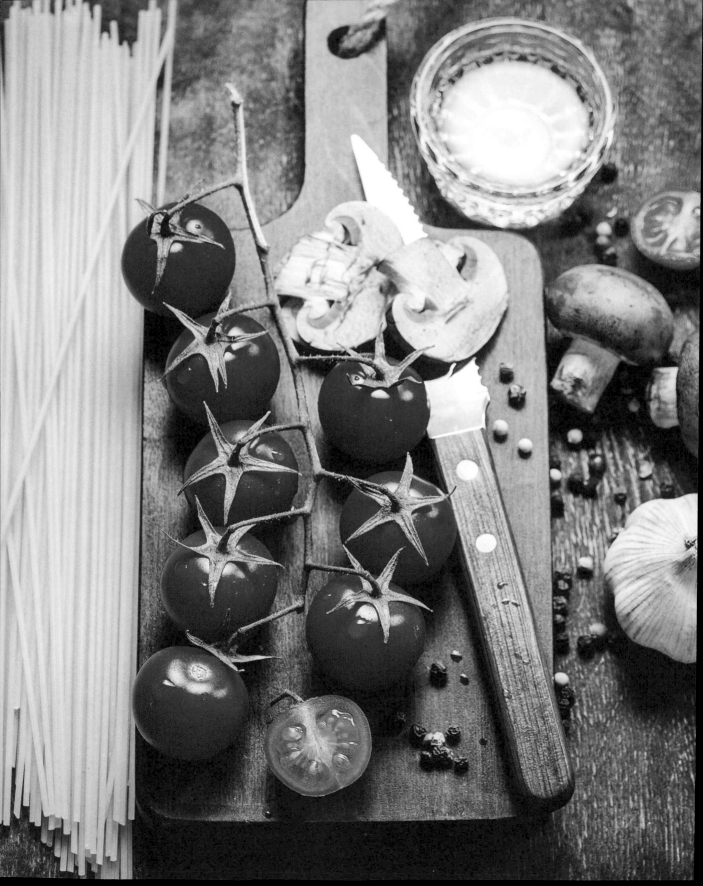

MAINS

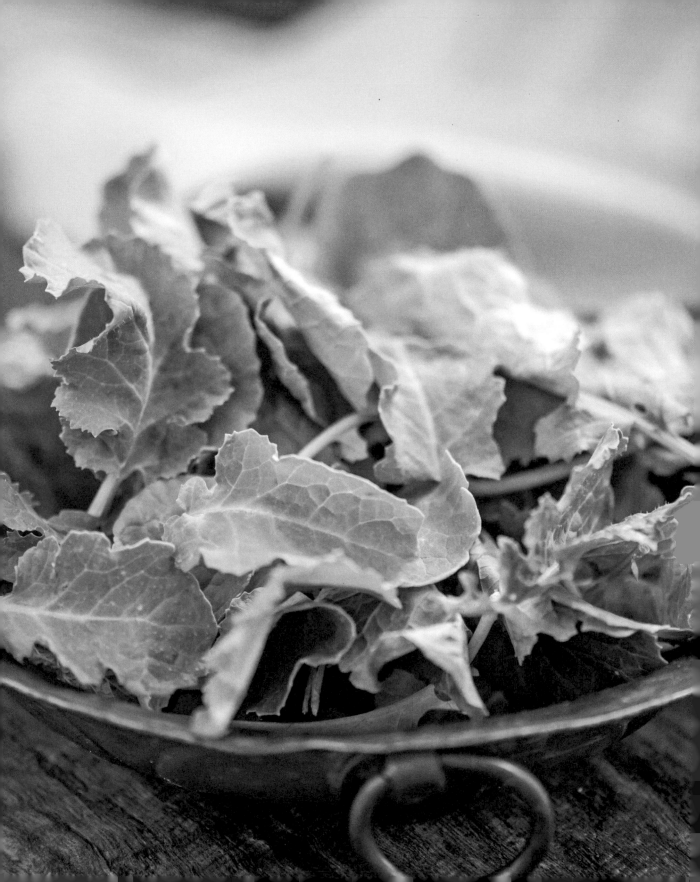

BABY KALE, ORANGE, WALNUTS & OLIVE SALAD WITH CITRUS VINAIGRETTE

Yield: Serves 6 / about 8 to 17 mg CBD per serving

Salads are one of my favorite things to make. I love to play with the textures, making a simple salad into an incredible meal. This one balances sweet and salty with some delightful crunch. This is a moderate CBD dose.

INGREDIENTS

For the citrus vinaigrette:
¼ cup (60 ml) fresh orange juice
1 tablespoon raw local honey
1 tablespoon (15 g) Dijon mustard
2 tablespoons (30 ml) extra-virgin
    olive oil
50 to 100 mg full-spectrum CBD oil
¼ teaspoon salt
¼ teaspoon freshly ground black pepper

For the salad:
4 seedless clementines or tangerines,
    peeled and segmented
¼ cup (25 g) walnuts, toasted and
    chopped
¼ cup (38.75 g) mixed pitted olives,
    chopped
5 ounces (140 g) baby kale

TIP *Buying clean baby kale will save lots of time and make this salad a cinch to whip up.*

METHOD OF PREPARATION:

1. To make the citrus vinaigrette: In a small bowl, whisk the orange juice, honey, and mustard until blended. Whisk in the olive oil and CBD oil until well combined and season with salt and pepper. Set aside.

2. To make the salad: In a large bowl combine the clementine segments, walnuts, olives, and baby kale; toss to distribute evenly.

3. Dress the salad and toss to combine.

SHRIMP SUMMER ROLLS
WITH SWEET CHILI SAUCE

Yield: Makes 8 summer rolls / 10 mg per serving

The summer roll is one of my greatest pleasures. The textures make me so happy. The colors make me smile and the sauce can be eaten with a spoon. These have a moderate CBD dose.

INGREDIENTS

For the sweet chili sauce:
½ cup(120 ml) rice vinegar
½ cup plus 2 tablespoons (125 g) organic unbleached sugar
¼ cup (60 ml) water
3 tablespoons (45 ml) fish sauce
2 tablespoons (30 ml) sherry or cooking sherry
3 garlic cloves, minced
1½ teaspoons to 1 tablespoon (5.6 g) red pepper flakes
1½ tablespoons (12 g) cornstarch dissolved in 3 tablespoons (45 ml) cold water
80 mg full-spectrum CBD oil

For the summer rolls:
12 medium shrimp, peeled, and deveined
8 (8¼-inch, or 20.6 cm) round rice paper wrappers
2 ounces (55 g) dried rice vermicelli, cooked according to the package directions and drained
½ cup (25 g) mung bean sprouts, rinsed and drained
24 small fresh mint leaves

16 fresh Thai basil leaves
8 cilantro sprigs
1 English cucumber, seeded and cut into ¼ x ¼ x 2-inch (0.6 x 0.6 x 5 cm) sticks
2 scallions, roots trimmed, halved, and cut into 3-inch (7.5 cm) lengths
4 Boston lettuce leaves, halved

METHOD OF PREPARATION:

❶ To prepare the shrimp: Bring a medium saucepan of water to a boil over high heat. Add the shrimp and cook for about 1 ½ minutes or until the shrimp are bright orange and just cooked. Drain the shrimp in a colander and run under cold water until they are cool. Halve shrimp lengthwise down the center. Cover and refrigerate.

❷ To make the sweet chili sauce: In a saucepan over high heat, combine the vinegar, sugar, water, fish sauce, sherry, garlic, and red pepper flakes. Bring the sauce to a rolling boil.

❸ Reduce the heat to medium and let boil for 10 minutes, or until reduced by half.

❹ Reduce the heat to low and stir in the cornstarch slurry. Cook for about 2 minutes, stirring occasionally, until the sauce thickens. Pour the sauce into a small bowl and let cool while you make the summer rolls.

❺ To make the summer rolls: Clear a work surface for rolling the summer rolls and have

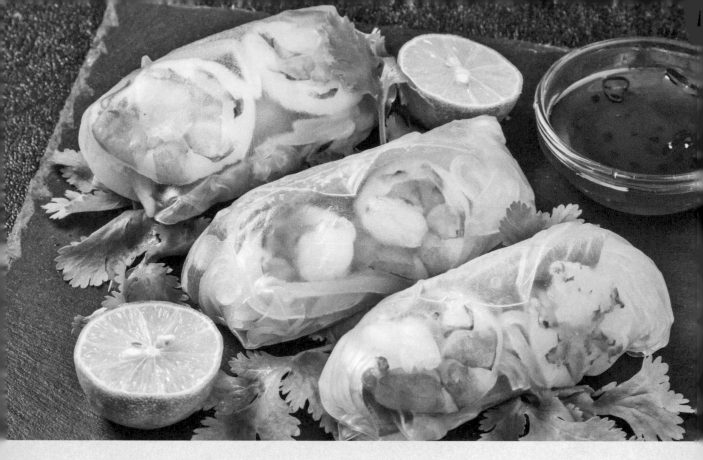

ready a baking pan roomy enough to hold the finished rolls in a single layer. Place all the filling ingredients in separate containers and arrange them around the work surface in the following order: rice paper wrappers, shrimp, rice noodles, bean sprouts, mint, basil, cilantro, cucumber, scallions, and lettuce.

6. Fill a wide shallow dish large enough to hold the rice paper wrappers with hot water. Evenly submerge one wrapper for about 30 seconds, or until it is soft and pliable. Remove from the water and place on the work surface.

7. Working quickly, layer a scant ¼ cup (44 g) of the rice noodles over the center of a rice wrapper, followed by a few bean sprouts, 3 mint leaves, 2 basil leaves, and 1 cilantro sprig. Place 3 to 4 cucumber sticks and 3 to 4 scallion pieces on either side of the noodle pile. Roll one piece of lettuce into a cigar shape and place it on top of the pile.

8. Fold the bottom half of the rice paper wrapper over the filling. Holding it firmly in place, fold the sides of the wrapper in. Pressing down to hold the folds in place, roll the entire pile up to close the top.

9. Turn the roll so the rice paper seam faces down, and the row of veggies faces up and place it in the baking pan. Cover the pan with a damp cloth and plastic wrap. Repeat to make the remaining rolls.

10. Whisk the CBD oil into the cooled sauce and serve with the summer rolls.

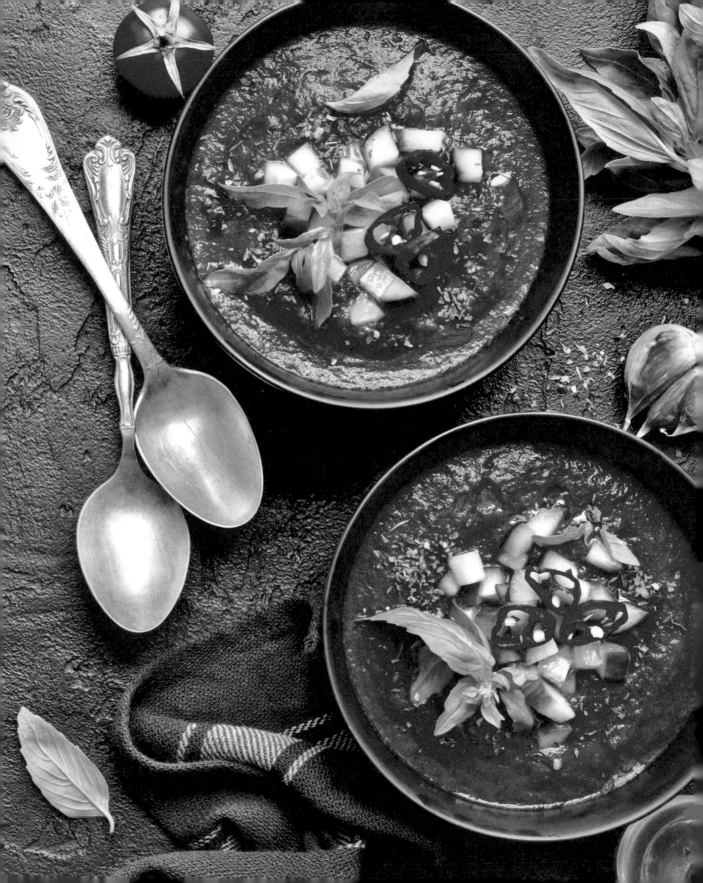

WATERMELON & TOMATO
GAZPACHO WITH CBD OLIVE OIL DRIZZLE

Yield: Serves 8 / 10 mg per serving

Gazpacho is one of those soups that I adore making in summer when both watermelon and tomatoes are at their peak. This refreshing cold soup is perfect for cooling off and relaxing during the hot months. This soup has a moderate dose of CBD.

INGREDIENTS

5 cups (750 g) chopped seedless watermelon
4 large beefsteak tomatoes, cored and roughly chopped
1 English cucumber, washed and chopped
4 basil sprigs, washed and leaves picked
4 cilantro sprigs, washed and leaves picked
¼ cup (48 g) baobab fruit powder
1½ teaspoons Maldon sea salt, plus more for seasoning
2 tablespoons (30 ml) sherry vinegar
6 tablespoons (90 ml) extra-virgin olive oil, divided
80 mg full-spectrum CBD oil
Diced cucumber, basil, and sliced mini peppers for topping

METHOD OF PREPARATION:

❶ In a food processor or blender, working in batches, combine the watermelon and tomatoes. Process until smooth and no chunks remain and transfer to a large bowl.

❷ In the same processor bowl, combine the cucumber, basil, cilantro, baobab powder, salt, and vinegar. With the processor running, slowly add 2 tablespoons (30 ml) of olive oil and continue to process until smooth. Transfer the mixture to the bowl with the watermelon and tomato juice. Refrigerate for at least 2 hours, or until ready to serve. (This may be done a day ahead and gives the flavors time to meld.)

❸ In a small bowl, whisk the remaining ¼ cup (60 ml) of olive oil and CBD oil.

❹ To serve, top the gazpacho with diced cucumber, basil, and sliced mini peppers. Season with salt, drizzle with the CBD-infused olive oil, toss the toppings and serve.

CHANA SAAG CHICKPEA SPINACH CURRY WITH CRISPY CBD CHICKPEAS

Yield: Serves 6 / 12.5 to 17 mg per serving

Indian food is so healing and nourishing to the body, with spices that naturally fight inflammation. This recipe has a moderate to high CBD dose.

INGREDIENTS

1 tablespoon (15 ml) olive oil

1-inch (2.5 cm) piece fresh ginger, peeled and grated

2 teaspoons ground cardamom

1 teaspoon ground cinnamon

1 teaspoon ground coriander

½ teaspoon ground turmeric

½ teaspoon chili powder

½ teaspoon garam masala

½ teaspoon sea salt

1 cup (160 g) finely chopped onion

6 garlic cloves, chopped

1 (15 ounces, or 425 g) can whole tomatoes, chopped

2 pounds (908 g) fresh baby spinach leaves

1½ cups (345 g) cashew yogurt or almond yogurt

2 (15 ounces, or 425 g each) cans chickpeas, rinsed and drained

1 (6 ounces, or 170 g) bag roasted salted crispy chickpeas

75 to 100 mg full-spectrum CBD oil

METHOD OF PREPARATION:

1. In a large nonstick sauté pan or skillet over medium heat, heat the olive oil. Add ginger, cardamom, cinnamon, coriander, turmeric, chili powder, garam masala, and salt. Cook, stirring, for 1 minute.

2. Increase the heat to medium-high. Add the onion and sauté until golden brown, about 3 minutes. Add the garlic and sauté for 30 seconds until fragrant.

3. Stir in the tomatoes and cook for 5 minutes, stirring frequently. Most of the liquid should evaporate and the mixture should be dark and caramelized.

4. Add half the spinach, stir, cover the pan, and cook for 1 minute. Remove the lid and add the remaining spinach. Re-cover the pan and cook for 1 minute more.

5. Once the spinach is wilted, transfer the mixture to a food processor. Add the yogurt and process until smooth.

6. Return the sauté pan to medium-low heat and transfer the spinach mixture to it. Add the chickpeas, turn the heat back up to a simmer, and cook for 10 minutes, stirring occasionally. Taste and adjust the seasonings.

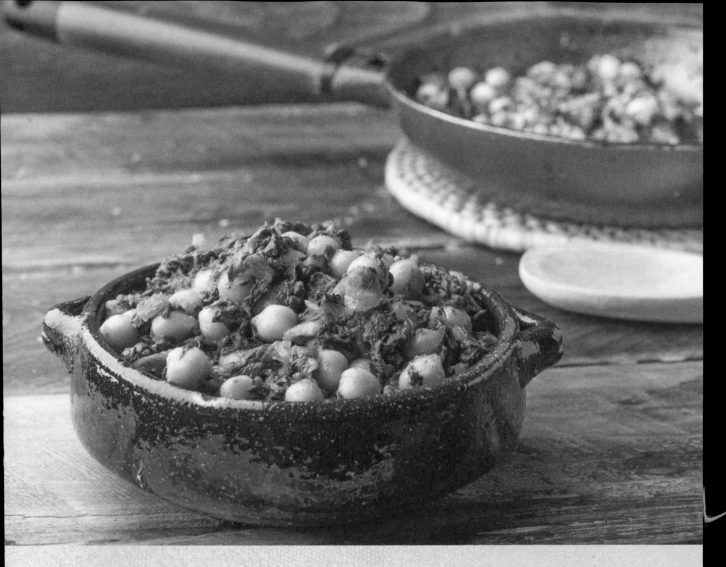

7   In a small sauté pan or skillet over low heat, warm the roasted chickpeas.

8   Add the CBD oil and toss to coat until well dispersed. Remove from the heat.

9   To serve, top the hot chana saag with the crispy chickpeas accompanied by naan, paratha, and brown basmati rice, as desired.

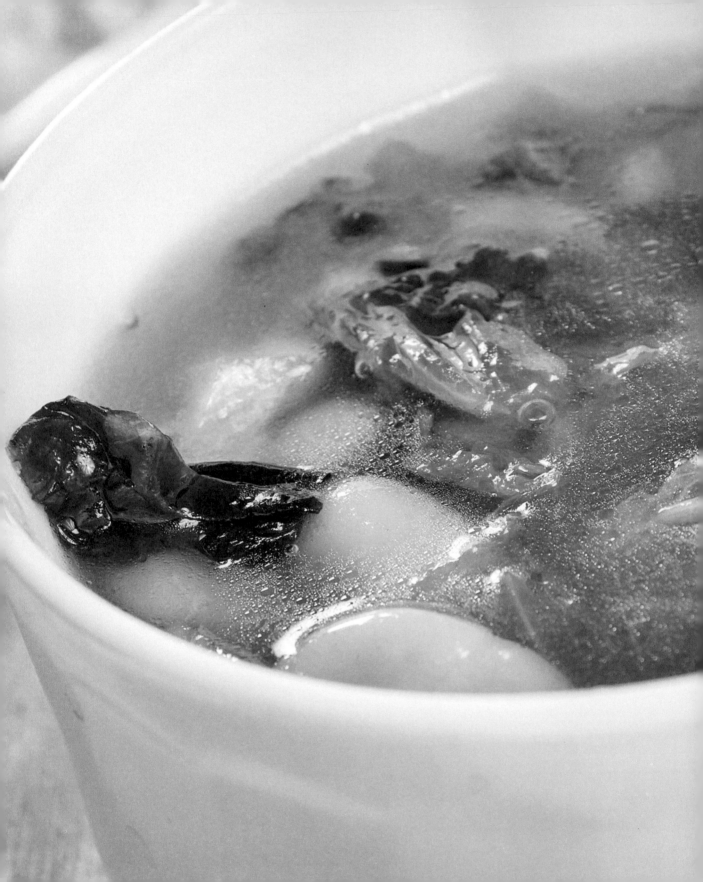

ESCAROLE & WHITE BEAN SOUP
WITH CBD INFUSED BROTH

Yield: Serves 6 / about 17 to 33 mg CBD per serving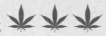

This hearty soup is a meal in and of itself. I adore the bitterness of escarole and the creaminess of white beans, add in a high dose of CBD and this soup is a great sleep aid, relaxation dinner, or recovery meal.

INGREDIENTS

1 tablespoon (15 ml) olive oil
1 medium onion, diced
2 large carrots, peeled and diced
2 celery stalks, diced
4 garlic cloves, minced
1 tablespoon (4 g) dried thyme
4 cups (200 g) washed, chopped
   escarole
2 (15.5 ounces, or 439 g each) cans
   cannellini beans, rinsed and drained
1 (1-inch, or 2.5 cm) piece Parmesan
   cheese rind
6 cups (1.4 L) good-quality vegetable
   broth
Sea salt
Freshly ground black pepper
100 to 200 mg full-spectrum CBD oil
¼ cup (25 g) freshly grated Parmesan
   cheese

METHOD OF PREPARATION:

1. In a large stockpot over medium heat, heat the olive oil until hot.

2. Add the onion, carrots, and celery. Sauté, stirring frequently, until translucent and a little caramelized, about 5 to 7 minutes.

3. Stir in the garlic and thyme. Cook, stirring, for 30 seconds.

4. Add the escarole. Cook for 4 to 5 minutes, stirring, until it wilts.

5. Add the cannellini beans, Parmesan rind, and vegetable broth and stir to combine. Taste and season with salt and pepper.

6. Bring the soup to a boil. Turn the heat to low and simmer for 30 minutes.

7. Remove the soup from the heat. Taste and season again—if needed—and stir in the CBD oil until well dispersed.

8. Serve with the grated Parmesan cheese for topping.

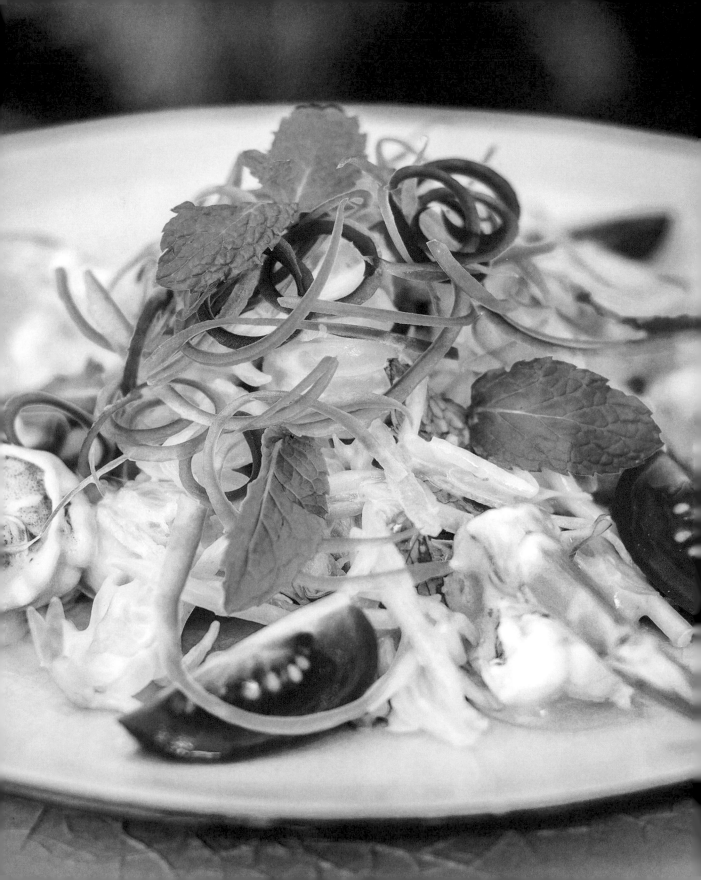

GREEN MANGO MUNG BEAN
NOODLE SALAD WITH CBD TOASTED COCONUT GRILLED SHRIMP

Yield: Serves 4 / 20 to 25 mg per serving

The flavors in this salad are so powerful that this will quickly become a favorite. The CBD dose is high, making this dish a perfect one to aid in a great night's sleep or a gentle post workout recovery.

INGREDIENTS

12 ounces (340 g) mung bean noodles
4 garlic cloves, peeled and minced
1 (4-inch, or 10 cm) piece fresh ginger, peeled and minced
2 tablespoons (40 g) chili sauce
½ cup (120 ml) fish sauce
⅓ cup (80 ml) water
½ cup (120 ml) fresh lime juice
½ cup (160 g) local raw honey
1 English cucumber, shredded
1 green mango, peeled and shredded
4 Napa cabbage leaves, thinly sliced
6 scallions, washed, root trimmed, and cut into long thin strips
1 jalapeño pepper, seeded and thinly sliced
⅓ cup (32 g) packed fresh mint leaves
⅓ cup (6 g) packed fresh cilantro leaves
⅓ cup (12 g) packed fresh Thai basil leaves
½ cup (40 g) unsweetened coconut, toasted
80 to 100 mg full-spectrum CBD oil
1 pound (454 g) large shrimp, peeled and deveined
1 tablespoon (15 ml) sesame oil
1 teaspoon sea salt

METHOD OF PREPARATION:

❶ In a large bowl, combine the noodles with enough very hot water to cover. Let stand for 5 minutes, or until very tender but not mushy. Drain in a colander and rinse with cold water.

❷ In a large bowl, whisk the garlic, ginger, chili sauce, fish sauce, water, lime juice, and honey.

❸ Add the drained noodles to the sauce along with the cucumber, mango, cabbage, scallions, jalapeño, mint, cilantro, and basil. Toss to coat and let sit for at least 10 minutes.

❹ In a small bowl, stir together the toasted coconut and CBD.

❺ Preheat a grill to high heat.

❻ In a medium bowl, toss together the shrimp, sesame oil, and salt.

❼ Once the grill is hot, place the shrimp on the grill rack and cook for 2 to 3 minutes, or until they turn pink and are slightly charred. Turn the shrimp and cook for 3 minutes on the second side. Remove to a plate and keep warm.

❽ When ready to serve, arrange the noodle salad on a platter, sprinkle with toasted coconut, and top with the grilled shrimp.

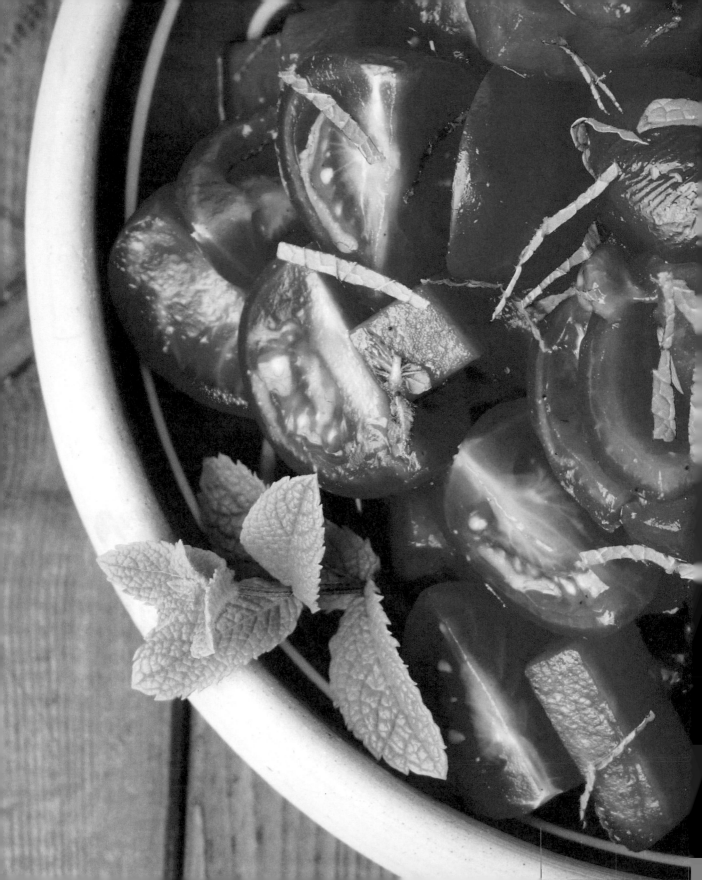

TOMATO, WATERMELON, BASIL & ARUGULA SALAD WITH CBD BALSAMIC DRESSING

Yield: Serves 4 / 25 mg per serving

This salad is my idea of summer on a plate. Make this when you have the meatiest, most-flavorful tomatoes and watermelon. This will not only ensure the most incredible flavor, but also the most nutrient-packed meal possible. This salad has a high CBD dose.

INGREDIENTS

4 heirloom tomatoes, different colors, washed, cored, and cut into bite-size pieces

2 cups (300 g) cubed (1-inch, or 2.5 cm pieces) baby seedless watermelon

1 cup (35 g) fresh basil leaves, washed and dried

4 cups (80 g) wild arugula, washed and dried

2 tablespoons (30 ml) extra-virgin olive oil

1½ tablespoons (23 ml) good-quality aged balsamic vinegar

100 mg full-spectrum CBD oil

1 teaspoon Maldon sea salt

¾ teaspoon freshly ground black pepper

METHOD OF PREPARATION:

1. Arrange the tomatoes on a large platter.

2. Add the watermelon cubes to the platter. Sprinkle with the basil and arugula. Set aside.

3. In a small bowl, whisk the olive oil, vinegar, and CBD oil and drizzle over the salad. Season with the salt and pepper.

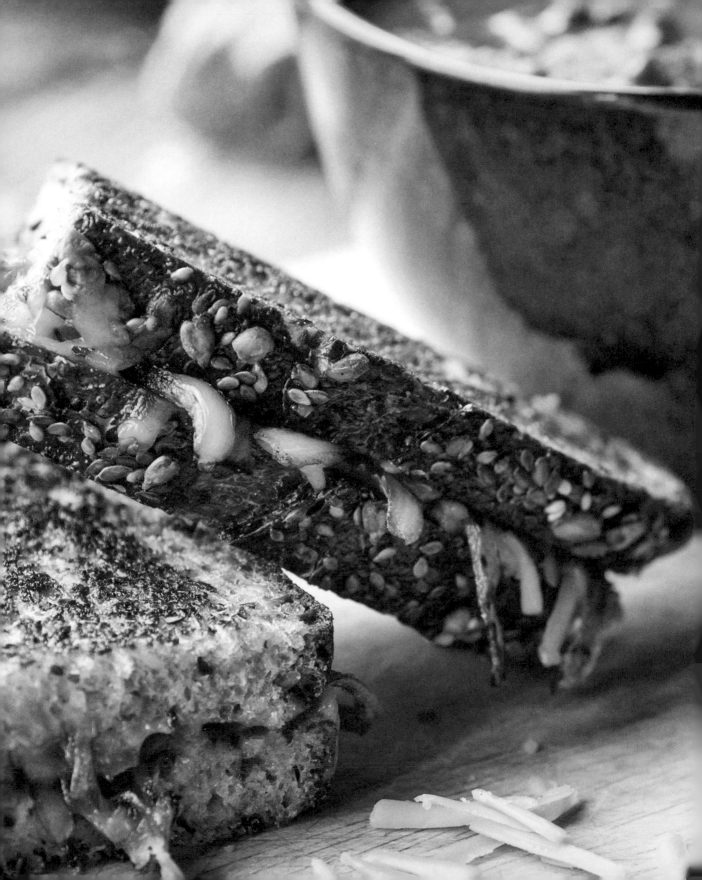

THE ULTIMATE VEGAN
—OR NOT—GRILLED CHEESE

Yield: Serves 2 / 20 to 25 mg per serving

Grilled cheese, whether you are plant based or not, is a serious comfort food. When I have a rough day or need a little extra comfort, a perfect grilled cheese with some tomato soup is one of my go tos. This sandwich is a perfect anxiety-reducing sleep aid and has a high CBD dose.

INGREDIENTS

2 tablespoons (28 g) dairy-free butter, such as Miyoko's
40 to 50 mg full-spectrum CBD oil
4 slices favorite bread (I love whole-wheat sourdough)
2 tablespoons (30 g) dairy-free scallion cream cheese, such as Kite Hill, or regular scallion cream cheese, at room temperature
4 slices dairy-free mature cheddar, such as Violife, or your favorite cheddar cheese
1 teaspoon Maldon sea salt

METHOD OF PREPARATION:

❶ Heat a large nonstick sauté pan or skillet over low heat. Add the butter to melt. Once the foam subsides, add the CBD oil.

❷ While the butter melts, prepare the sandwiches. Divide the cream cheese between two bread slices, smearing it over. Top each with 2 slices of cheese and top the sandwiches with the remaining slices of bread.

❸ Add the sandwiches to the pan, coating one side in the butter. Flip the sandwiches to the other side and cover the pan with a glass lid. Cook for 5 to 7 minutes, or until the sandwiches are golden and toasted and the cheese has begun to melt. Flip the sandwiches, re-cover the pan, and cook for 5 to 7 minutes more, or until browned and the cheese has melted.

❹ Transfer the sandwiches to a cutting board, cut on the diagonal, and sprinkle with salt.

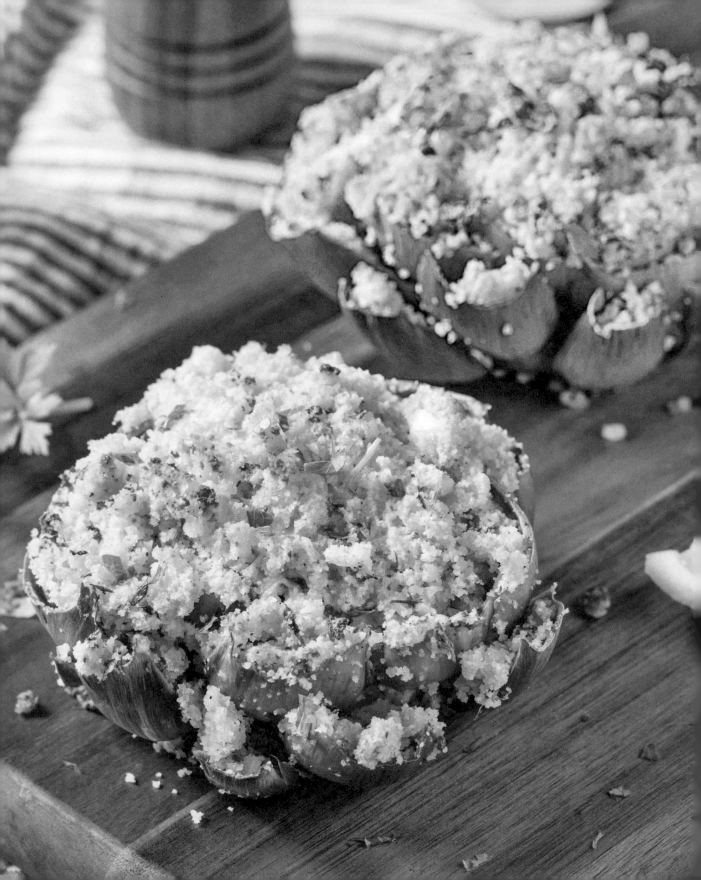

ITALIAN STUFFED ARTICHOKES
WITH CBD-INFUSED LEMON SAUCE

Yield: Serves 4 / 20 to 25 mg per serving

Growing up, Italian stuffed artichokes were my favorite food. In fact, from the time I was 4 until now, they have been my birthday meal! I find them so unique in the amount of work that goes into eating them and how greatly you are rewarded when you come to the heart. This special dish has a high CBD dose and is a perfect one to relax and unwind.

INGREDIENTS

For the artichokes:
1 cup (115 g) Italian-style breadcrumbs
½ cup (50 g) cubed Pecorino Romano
   cheese
4 garlic cloves, thinly sliced
4 large globe artichokes
4 teaspoons (20 ml) extra-virgin olive oil
½ teaspoon kosher salt
Freshly ground black pepper

For the CBD-infused lemon sauce:
1 cup (230 g) plain almond yogurt or
   cashew yogurt
¼ cup (60 ml) fresh lemon juice
1 tablespoon (6 g) lemon zest
4 dashes hot sauce
80 to 100 mg full-spectrum CBD oil
1 teaspoon sea salt
½ teaspoon freshly ground black pepper

METHOD OF PREPARATION:

1. To make the artichokes: Bring a large stockpot filled one-quarter of the way with water to a boil over high heat. Insert a steamer.

2. In a small bowl, stir together the breadcrumbs, Pecorino Romano cheese, and garlic. Set aside.

3. To clean the artichokes, cut off about ½ inch (1 cm) of the prickly tops. Cut off the stems so a flat surface on the bottom of the artichoke remains.

4. Pull the leaves away from the artichoke, creating pockets for stuffing. Add the breadcrumb mixture, making sure to spread it all around.

5. Drizzle the artichokes with olive oil and season with salt and pepper. Place them into the steamer basket and cover. Turn the heat to medium and steam for 1 hour, checking periodically to make sure the water level does not need to be replenished.

6. To make the CBD-infused lemon sauce: While the artichokes cook, in a medium bowl, whisk the yogurt, lemon juice, lemon zest, hot sauce, CBD oil, salt, and pepper. Set aside until ready to serve.

7. Serve the artichokes warm with the dipping sauce.

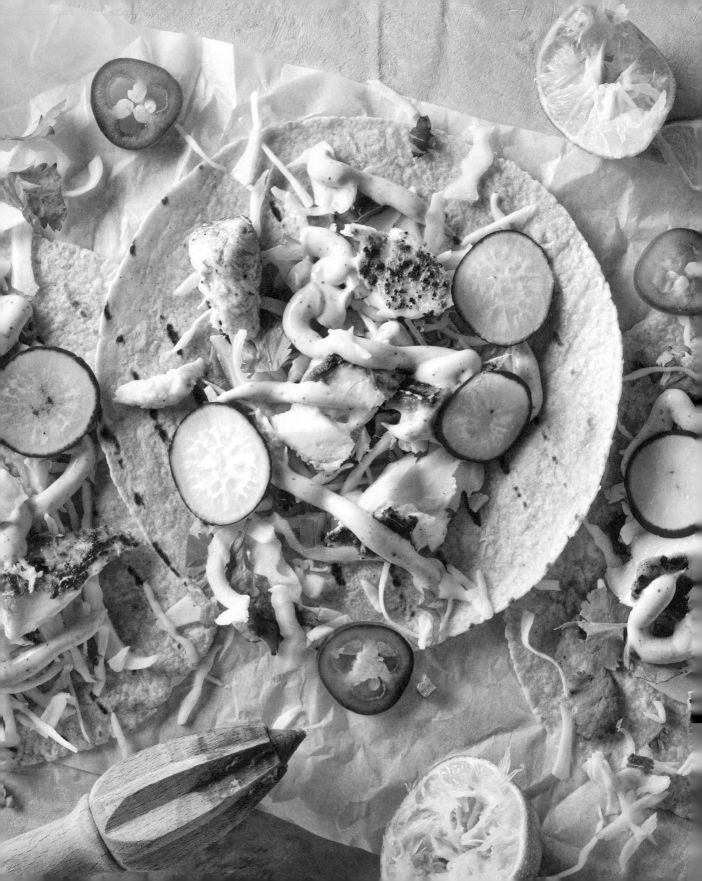

FISH TACOS
WITH CABBAGE & RADISHES

Yield: Serves 4 / 25 mg CBD per serving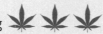

Tacos are one of my passions. This simple recipe is full of flavor and bursting with textures and spices. This recipe has a high CBD dose.

INGREDIENTS

8 soft taco-size tortillas, Ezekiel, whole wheat, corn, or white, wrapped in aluminum foil
1 teaspoon avocado oil
1 teaspoon ground cumin
1 teaspoon chili powder
Juice of 1 lime
½ teaspoon sea salt
4 (4 ounces, or 115 g each) red snappers, halved lengthwise
1 cup (70 g) thinly sliced green or red cabbage
½ cup (58 g) thinly sliced radishes
100 mg full-spectrum CBD oil
2 avocados, peeled, pitted, and sliced

TIP *You can easily make this with tofu, shrimp, or other type of firm, white fish.*

METHOD OF PREPARATION:

1. Preheat the oven to 400°F (200°C).

2. Place the foil-wrapped tortillas in the oven for 10 minutes to warm.

3. While the tortillas warm, in a large bowl, stir together the avocado oil, cumin, chili powder, lime juice, and salt. Add the fish and turn to coat well. Let sit for 5 to 10 minutes.

4. In a medium bowl, toss together the cabbage and radishes and set aside.

5. Heat a large sauté pan or skillet over medium-high heat. Add the marinated fish and sear for 3 minutes per side. Remove from the heat and drizzle the fish with CBD oil.

6. To serve, place a piece of fish on each warmed tortilla, top with cabbage, radishes, and sliced avocado.

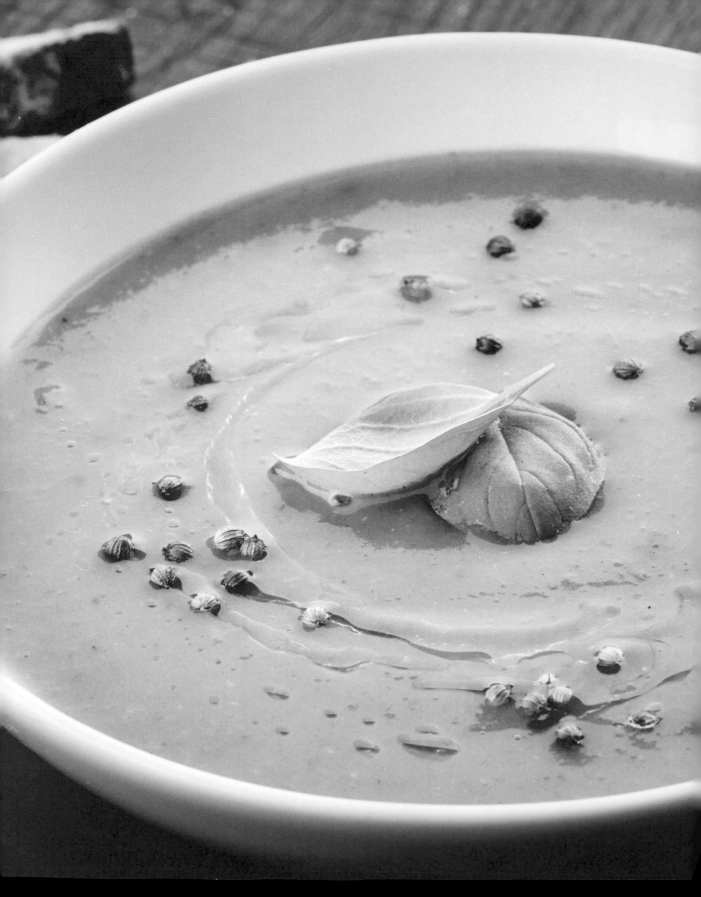

MISO, YAM, CARROT & GINGER
CBD RECOVERY SOUP

Yield: Serves 6 / 20 to 30 mg per serving

This recovery soup is one I developed for the athletes in my life. It nourishes the body on so many levels, pre and probiotics, stomach soother, inflammation buster— it truly is medicine in a bowl. This soup has a high CBD dose.

INGREDIENTS

2 tablespoons (30 ml) avocado oil
1 sweet onion, chopped
1 (2-inch, or 5 cm) piece fresh ginger, peeled and chopped
3 garlic cloves, roughly chopped
2 cups (220 g) peeled, chopped Japanese yam
1 ½ cups (195 g) peeled, chopped carrot
2 quarts (1.9 L) good-quality vegetable broth
½ cup (125 g) red miso paste
2 tablespoons (30 ml) tamari
120 to 180 mg full-spectrum CBD oil

TIP *If you can't find red miso, white or yellow miso will work fine. The end product will be a little less robust in flavor, but still delicious!*

METHOD OF PREPARATION:

❶   In a large stockpot over medium heat, heat the avocado oil. Add the onion, ginger, and garlic. Sauté for 5 minutes.

❷   Stir in the yam, carrot, and vegetable broth. Turn the heat to high and bring the mixture to a boil. Reduce the heat to medium-low and simmer for 30 to 40 minutes, or until the yam and carrot are tender.

❸   Remove the soup from the heat and stir in the miso paste and tamari.

❹   Working in batches, transfer the soup to a high-powered blender and purée until smooth and creamy. Transfer the soup back to the stockpot and whisk in the CBD oil to disperse evenly.

❺   Serve as a workout recovery soup.

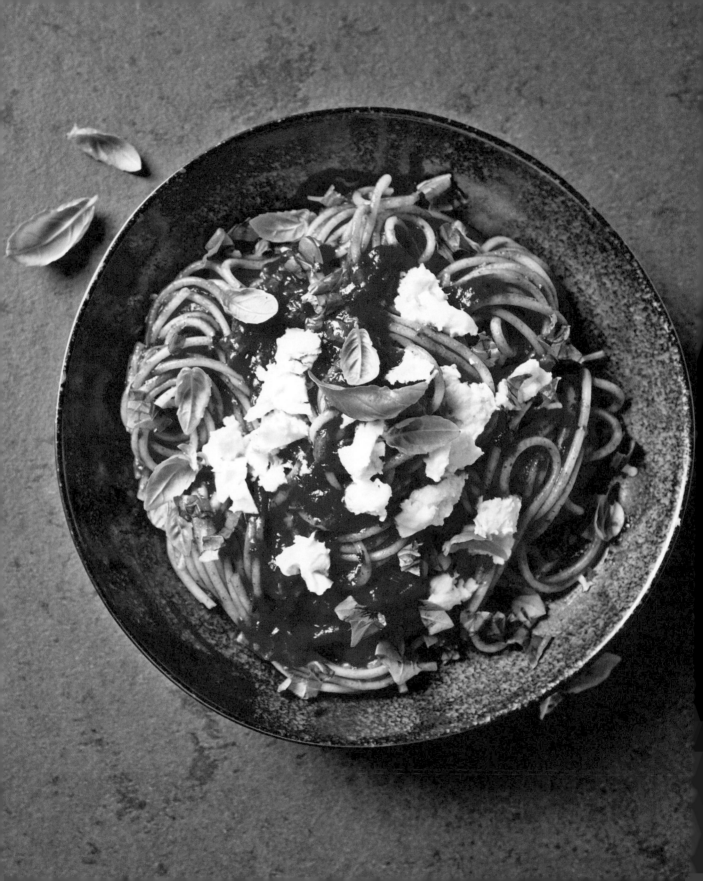

CBD-INFUSED
PASTA MARGARITA

Yield: Serves 6 / 20 to 30 mg per serving

This simple tomato sauce is only to be made when you have the most flavorful summer tomatoes, otherwise it's just not worth it. That said, with the ripest most flavorful tomatoes, this super simple pasta sauce will blow you away!

INGREDIENTS

½ teaspoon sea salt, plus more for the pasta water

1 pound (454 g) fresh linguine

¼ cup (60 ml) extra-virgin olive oil

6 garlic cloves, minced

2 pounds (908 g) heirloom tomatoes or very good ripe tomatoes, seeded and chopped

½ cup (20 g) basil, roughly chopped

8 ounces (225 g) buffalo mozzarella, diced

Freshly ground black pepper

120 to 180 mg full-spectrum CBD oil

TIP *This pasta is wonderful served warm, but equally as excellent the next day cold.*

METHOD OF PREPARATION:

❶ Bring a large pot of salted water to a boil over high heat. Add the linguine and cook according to the package directions. Drain and reserve 1 cup of cooking liquid.

❷ In a large sauté pan or skillet over medium heat, heat the olive oil. Add the garlic and sauté for 30 seconds.

❸ Add the tomatoes, basil, and mozzarella. Turn off the heat.

❹ Add the cooked pasta and reserved cooking liquid. Gently toss to combine. Season with salt, pepper, and the CBD oil.

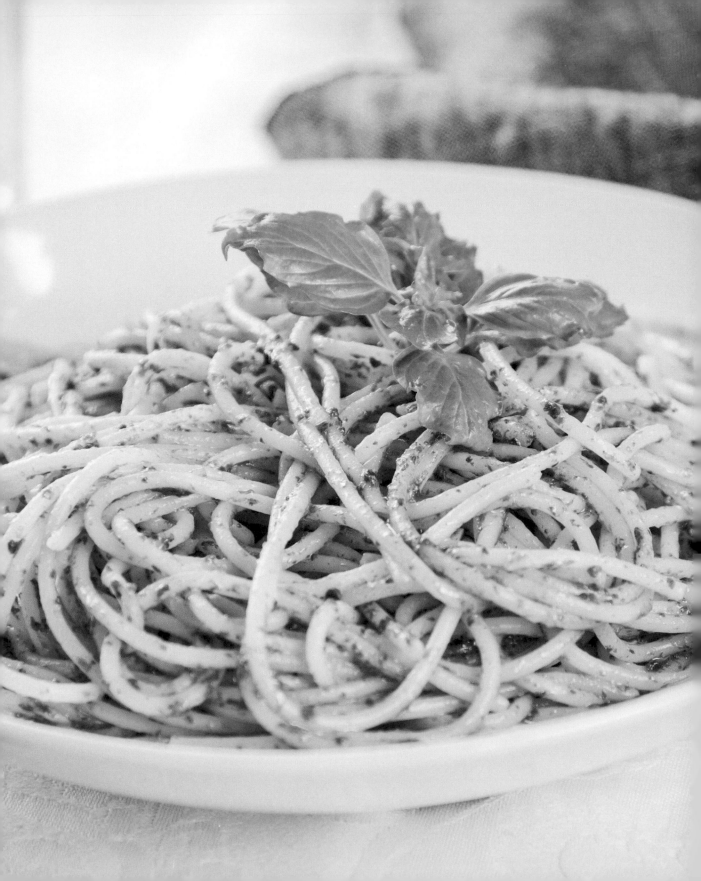

SPAGHETTI
WITH CBD PISTACHIO PESTO

Yield: Serves 4 / 20 to 30 mg per serving

Who doesn't love pesto? And this one made with pistachios is more decadent than the traditional pine nut method. Pasta is always a great pre- and post-workout meal and this one is packed with healing abilities. This is a high CBD dose.

INGREDIENTS

½ cup (64 g) shelled pistachios
⅓ cup (38 g) chunked Parmesan cheese
    or vegan Parmesan
4 garlic cloves, peeled
2 cups (70 g) packed fresh basil leaves
10 ounces (280 g) fresh baby spinach
    leaves
½ cup (60 to 120 ml) water, divided
⅓ cup (80 ml) extra-virgin olive oil
¼ teaspoon kosher salt
Freshly ground black pepper
1 pound (454 g) favorite spaghetti,
    cooked according to the package
    directions, drained, and 1 cup
    (240 ml) cooking liquid reserved
80 to 120 mg full-spectrum CBD oil

METHOD OF PREPARATION:

1. In a food processor, combine the pistachios, Parmesan cheese, and garlic. Pulse until finely chopped.

2. Add the basil, spinach, and ¼ cup (60 ml) of water. Pulse until smooth. If a thinner consistency is desired, add the remaining ¼ cup (60 ml) of water

3. With the processor running, slowly add the olive oil. Taste and season with salt and pepper.

4. To serve, in a large sauté pan or skillet over medium heat, combine the cooked pasta, pesto, and reserved cooking liquid. Sauté for 2 minutes, or until hot and creamy.

5. Remove the pan from the heat and stir in the CBD oil until well dispersed.

FALAFEL
WITH GARLICKY CBD TAHINI SAUCE

Yield: Serves 4 / 20 to 40 mg per serving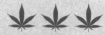

Falafel, protein rich and oh so flavorful, this delicious nutrient-packed meal is a great pre or post workout energy boost. The CBD dose is high.

INGREDIENTS

For the falafel:
2 whole-wheat pita bread rounds, halved and wrapped in aluminum foil
1 (15 ounces, or 425 g) can chickpeas, rinsed and drained
2 garlic cloves, crushed
½ cup (30 g) fresh parsley leaves
¼ cup (40 g) diced sweet onion
1 tablespoon (15 g) tahini
1½ teaspoons ground cumin
1 teaspoon fresh lemon juice
½ teaspoon sea salt
½ teaspoon red pepper flakes
½ teaspoon dried mint
3½ tablespoons (27 g) all-purpose flour
1 teaspoon baking powder
2 cups (480 ml) avocado oil

For the tahini sauce:
3 tablespoons (45 g) tahini
60 to 160 mg full-spectrum CBD oil
2 tablespoons (40 g) honey
2 tablespoons (30 ml) water
1 teaspoon soy sauce
1 teaspoon fresh lemon juice
½ teaspoon minced garlic
1 tablespoon (4 g) chopped fresh parsley leaves
1 tablespoon (6 g) chopped fresh mint leaves
1 teaspoon salt

For serving:
1 large tomato, sliced
1 head romaine lettuce, washed and leaves separated
½ cup (120 g) sliced cucumber

METHOD OF PREPARATION:

❶ Preheat the oven to 200°F (93°C).

❷ Place the foil-wrapped bread in the oven.

❸ In a food processor, combine the chickpeas, garlic, parsley, onion, tahini, cumin, lemon juice, salt, red pepper flakes, and mint. Pulse until a rough paste forms. Add the flour and baking powder and pulse until well combined.

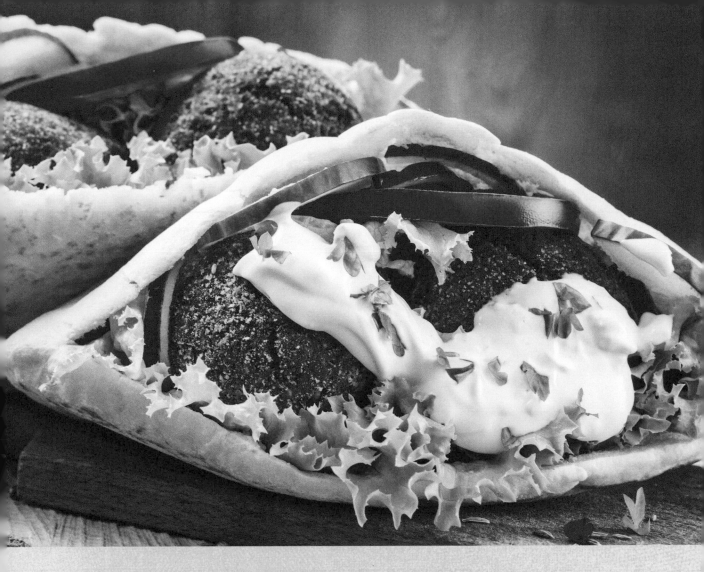

4 In a large skillet over medium high-heat, heat the avocado oil for 2 to 3 minutes. Working in batches, carefully drop heaping tablespoonfuls of the falafel batter into the hot oil. Fry for 1½ to 2 minutes until golden. Flip and fry the other side. Remove to a paper towel–lined plate to drain. Repeat with the remaining falafel. Keep the cooked falafel warm in the oven until ready to serve.

5 To make the tahini sauce: In a medium bowl, combine the tahini, CBD oil, honey, water, soy sauce, lemon juice, and garlic. Whisk until smooth. Stir in the parsley, mint, and salt and refrigerate until ready to use. Bring to room temperature before serving.

6 To serve, place four falafel inside half a warmed pita. Stuff with sliced tomato, romaine lettuce, and sliced cucumber and drizzle with tahini sauce.

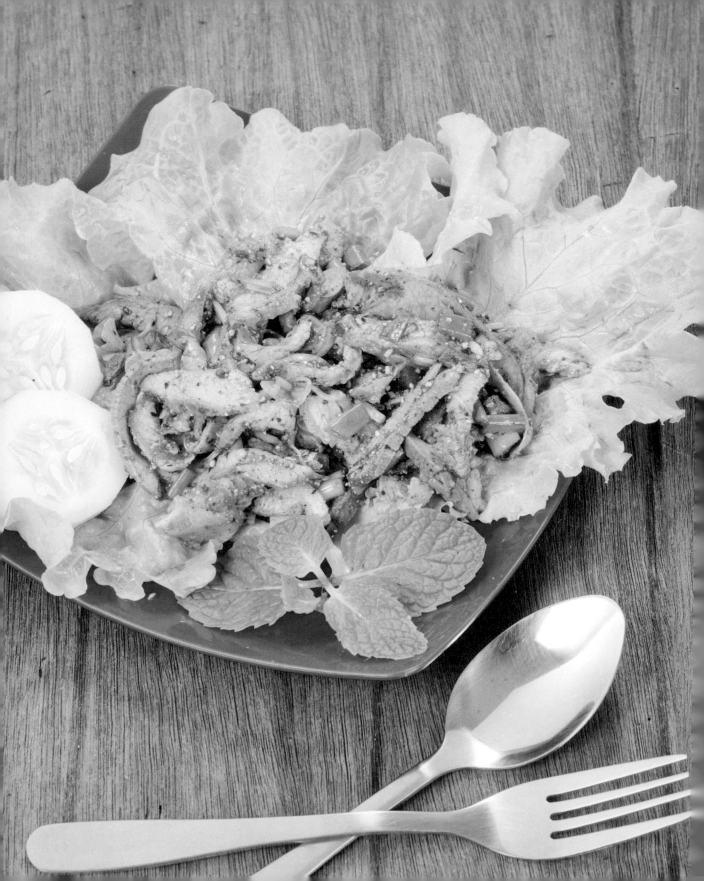

GROUND CHICKEN
OR VEGETABLE PROTEIN LARB
WITH MINT & THAI BASIL IN LETTUCE CUPS

Yield: Serves 4 / 25 to 50 mg CBD per serving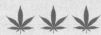

Laarb is one of my favorite Thai dishes. Typically, it is made with ground chicken or pork, this one uses TVP or textured vegetable protein, but feel free to use what you love! The balance of sweet, spicy, sour, and salty is what makes Thai cuisine so special. Add in a high dose of CBD and this dish is a wonderful and relaxing entrée.

INGREDIENTS

2 tablespoons (23 g) basmati rice
100 to 200 mg full-spectrum CBD oil
¼ cup (60 ml) fresh lime juice
1-pound (454 g) ground chicken or turkey, half dark meat, half white meat, or dehydrated textured vegetable protein (TVP)
1 teaspoon toasted sesame oil
2 shallots, thinly sliced
½ teaspoon red pepper flakes
¼ cup (60 ml) fish sauce
2 tablespoons (2 g) chopped fresh cilantro
2 tablespoons (5 g) chopped fresh Thai basil
2 tablespoons (12 g) chopped fresh mint
2 scallions, chopped
1 head iceberg lettuce, leaves removed and kept whole, washed and dried
2 limes, quartered

METHOD OF PREPARATION:

1. In a small sauté pan or skillet over medium heat, toast the rice for 3 minutes, or until golden brown. Some rice will pop like popcorn. Transfer the toasted rice to a mortar and use the pestle to grind the rice until it resembles breadcrumbs. Alternatively, transfer the rice to a spice grinder and grind. Stir in the CBD oil and set aside.

2. In a medium bowl, mix together the lime juice and ground meat or TVP. Let sit while you cook the shallots.

3. In a large nonstick sauté pan or wok, over medium-high heat, heat the sesame oil. Add the shallots and sauté until lightly browned, about 3 minutes.

4. Add the marinated ground meat or TVP and red pepper flakes. Cook for 5 minutes, stirring occasionally, or until the meat is crumbled and cooked through.

5. Remove from the heat. Stir in the fish sauce, cilantro, basil, mint, scallions, and ground toasted rice. Transfer the mixture to a serving dish.

6. To serve, arrange the lettuce leaves and lime wedges on a platter. Allow diners to make their own laarb lettuce wraps and season with lime juice, as desired.

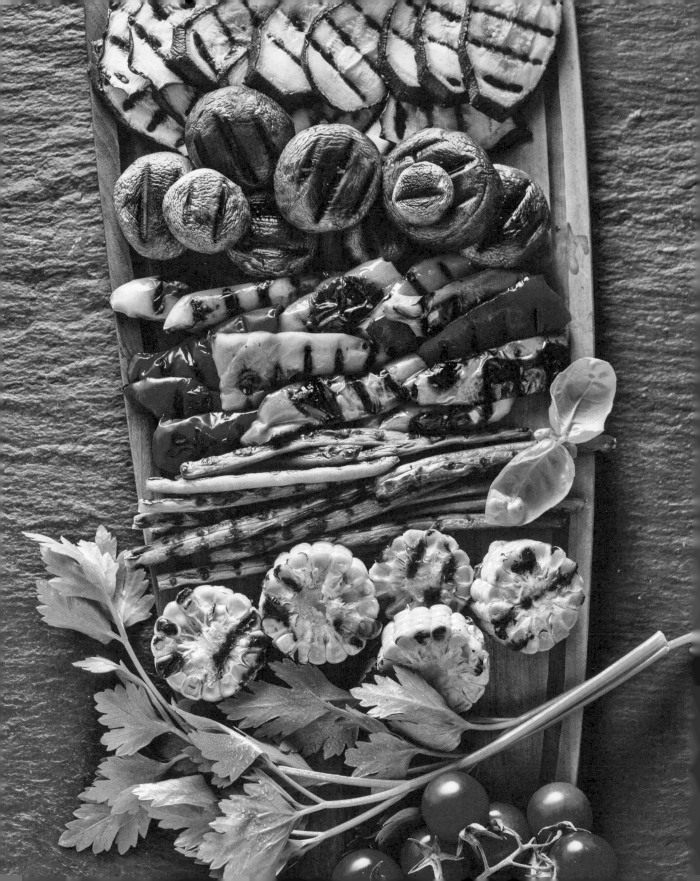

SIDE DISHES

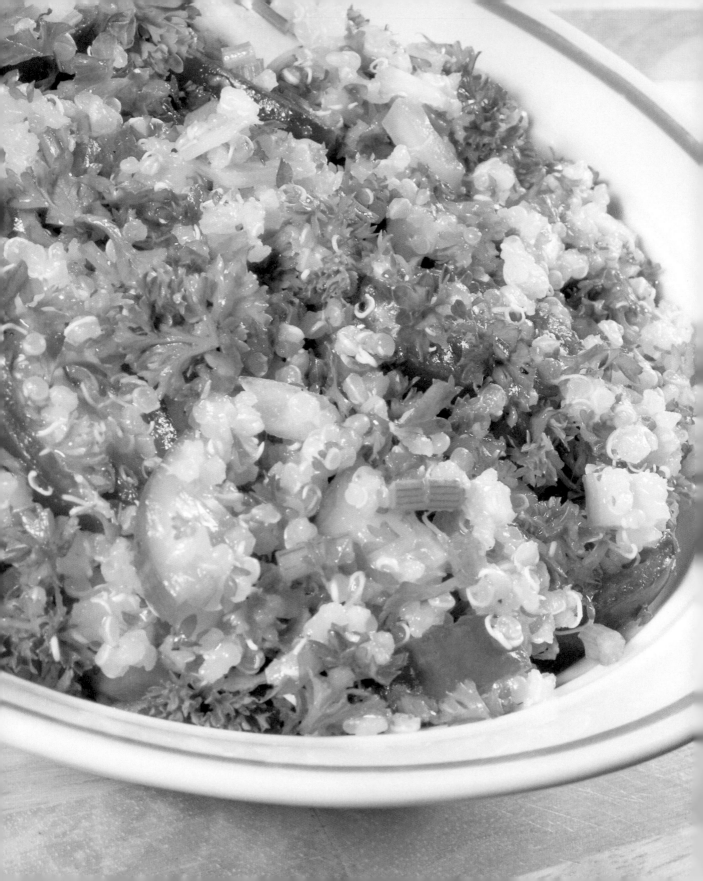

CBD QUINOA
TABBOULEH

Yield: Serves 8 / 3 to 4 mg per serving

Tabbouleh is such a bright side dish, filled with protein-rich quinoa, fresh herbs, and lemon juice. You want to use the best ingredients because they are simply showcased in this one. This dish has a low dose of CBD.

INGREDIENTS

1 cup (184 g) red or white quinoa, rinsed well

2 cups (480 ml) vegetable broth or water

3 bunches fresh parsley, washed and chopped

¼ cup (24 g) fresh mint, washed and chopped

4 scallions, washed, roots trimmed, and chopped

2 large tomatoes, diced

1 English cucumber, seeded and chopped

1½ teaspoons sea salt

¼ teaspoon freshly ground black pepper

⅓ cup (80 ml) fresh lemon juice

¼ cup (60 ml) extra-virgin olive oil

24 to 32 mg full-spectrum CBD oil

TIP *Keep a glass container full of cooked quinoa at the ready for Buddha bowls, salads, or anything really. Having cooked quinoa ready makes this side dish a snap.*

METHOD OF PREPARATION:

❶ In a medium saucepan over high heat, combine the quinoa and broth. Bring to a boil, cover the pan, reduce the heat to low, and simmer for 15 minutes. Turn off the heat and let the quinoa steam, covered, for 5 minutes. Transfer to a large bowl and let cool.

❷ Add the parsley, mint, scallions, tomatoes, cucumber, salt, pepper, lemon juice, olive oil, and CBD oil to the cooled quinoa. Toss well to combine. Taste and adjust the seasonings, as needed. Serve at room temperature.

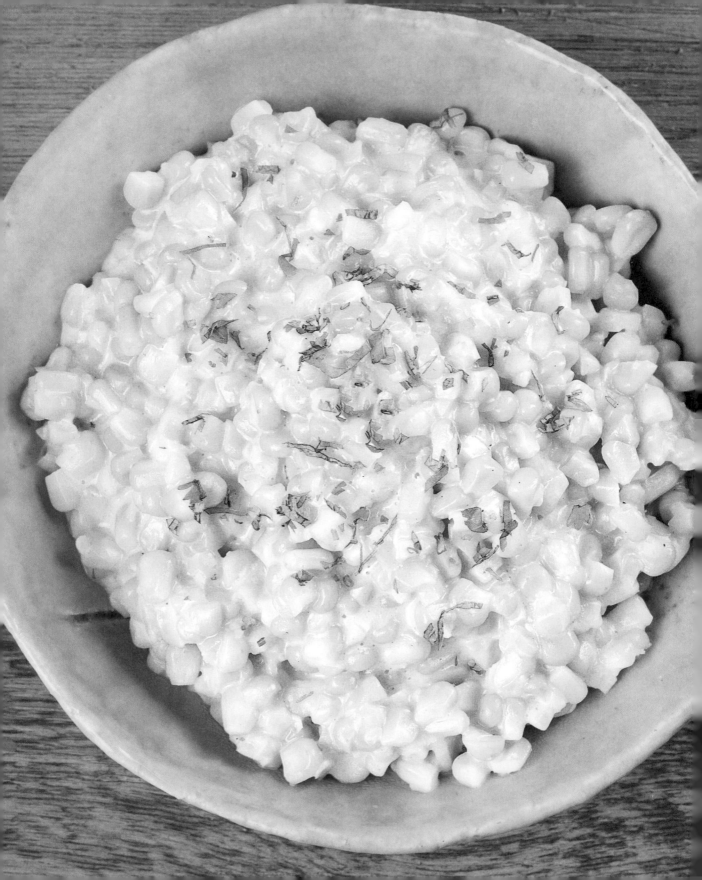

EASY "CREAMED" CORN
WITH THYME, ROSEMARY & CBD

Yield: Serves 4 / 5 to 10 mg CBD

I am a southern girl at heart but also a lover of fresh and healthy vegetables. That's quite a conundrum! Creamed corn is typically a heavy dish, but I've lightened it considerably without losing any of the flavor. Best made when corn is at its peak season. This dish has a low to moderate CBD dose.

INGREDIENTS

1 tablespoon (15 ml) olive oil
6 ears corn, shucked and kernels cut
    from the cobs
½ cup (120 ml) unsweetened hemp milk
½ cup (115 g) dairy-free scallion cream
    cheese, such as Kite Hill, or another
    favorite brand
1 tablespoon (2.4 g) fresh thyme leaves,
    chopped
1 tablespoon (1.7 g) fresh rosemary
    leaves, chopped
20 to 40 mg full-spectrum CBD oil
Sea salt
Freshly ground black pepper

METHOD OF PREPARATION:

❶ In a large sauté pan or skillet over medium-high heat, heat the olive oil. Add the corn kernels, cover the pan, and cook until light brown and tender, about 10 minutes.

❷ Transfer the corn to a food processor. While pulsing, slowly add the milk and cream cheese and process until creamy and thick. Add the thyme, rosemary, and CBD oil and season with salt and pepper. Pulse to combine.

❸ Return the corn mixture to the sauté pan and simmer over low heat for 5 minutes to warm.

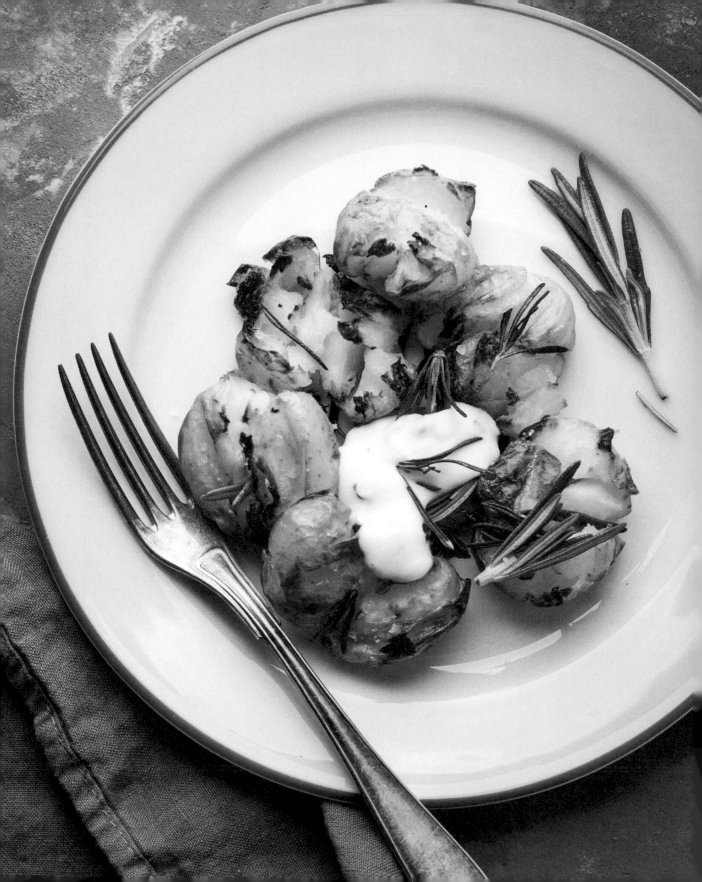

GRILLED & SMASHED
NEW POTATOES WITH CBD CRÈME FRAÎCHE

Yield: Serves 4 / 5 mg per serving

These potatoes are going to become a grill-out favorite. They are so simple and so delicious!

INGREDIENTS

2 pounds (908 g) baby creamer potatoes
2 tablespoons (30 ml) olive oil
1 tablespoon (18 g) kosher salt
1 tablespoon (6 g) freshly ground black
    pepper
½ cup (115 g) crème fraîche
20 mg full-spectrum CBD oil
1 sprig fresh rosemary, chopped, for
    garnish

TIP *To make these plant-based, nix the crème fraîche and opt for an almond based scallion cream cheese, such as Kite Hill.*

METHOD OF PREPARATION:

❶ Preheat the grill to medium heat.

❷ In a large bowl, combine the potatoes, olive oil, salt, and pepper and toss to coat. Wrap the seasoned potatoes in aluminum foil and seal closed or place them in a grill basket.

❸ Place the potatoes on the grill, close the lid, and grill for 1 hour, flipping the foil package halfway through the grilling time. The potatoes are done when a knife inserted into them comes out easily. Transfer the potatoes to a cutting board.

❹ Using the bottom of a heavy drinking glass, flatten each potato. Transfer them to a platter.

❺ In a small bowl, stir together the crème fraîche and CBD oil, mixing well. Pour the sauce over the smashed potatoes and sprinkle with the rosemary.

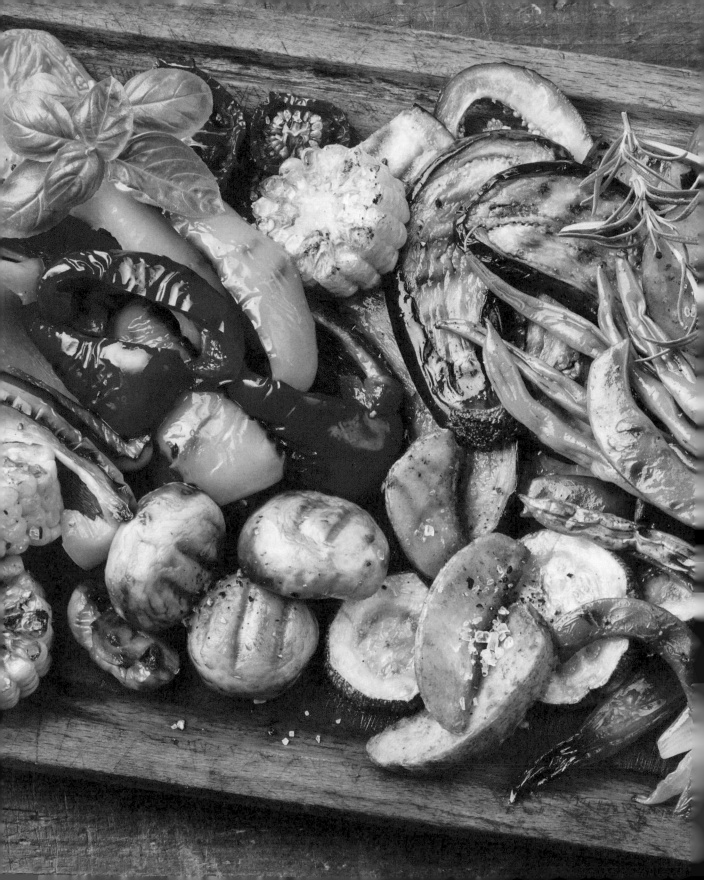

GRILLED VEGETABLES
WITH GREEN TAHINI SAUCE

Yield: Serves 4 / 5 to 10 mg per serving

There is something so satisfying about grilled vegetables. The flavor imparted on them is like no other. This simple side dish is elegant and a great addition to any meal. This dish has a low to moderate CBD dose.

INGREDIENTS

For the vegetables:
3 red, yellow, or orange bell peppers, seeded and halved
3 yellow squash, sliced lengthwise into ½-inch (1 cm)-thick rectangles
3 zucchinis, sliced lengthwise into ½-inch (1 cm)-thick rectangles
20 cremini mushrooms, wiped clean
1 bunch asparagus, woody ends trimmed
12 scallions, roots cut off and cleaned
¼ cup (60 ml) olive oil
1 tablespoon (18 g) kosher salt
1 tablespoon (6 g) freshly ground black pepper

Ingredients for green tahini sauce:
3 garlic cloves, peeled
¾ cup (12 g) fresh cilantro
¾ cup (45 g) fresh parsley
1 teaspoon ground cumin
2 teaspoons kosher salt
1 cup (240 g) tahini
¼ cup (60 ml) fresh lemon juice
20 to 40 mg full-spectrum CBD oil

METHOD OF PREPARATION:

1. To make the vegetables: Preheat the grill to medium heat.

2. Brush all the vegetables with olive oil to lightly coat. Sprinkle with salt and pepper.

3. Working in batches, grill the vegetables until tender and lightly charred all over, about 8 to 10 minutes for the bell peppers, 7 minutes for the squash, zucchini, and mushrooms, and 4 minutes for the asparagus and scallions. Transfer the grilled vegetables to a platter.

4. To make the green tahini sauce: In a high-powered blender, combine all the sauce ingredients and purée until smooth and creamy.

5. To serve, drizzle the grilled vegetables with the tahini sauce and serve hot or at room temperature.

SPINACH-ARTICHOKE
GRATIN WITH CBD

Yield: Serves 6 / 5 to 10 mg per serving

A very elegant side dish that will make any special occasion meal excel. This dish has a low to moderate CBD dose.

INGREDIENTS

2 (10 ounces, or 280 g each) packages chopped frozen spinach, thawed

1 (10 ounce, or 280 g) package frozen artichoke hearts in water, thawed

4 tablespoons (30 ml) olive oil, divided

2 cups (320 g) diced yellow onion

1 teaspoon kosher salt

2 tablespoons (15.5 g) all-purpose flour

½ cup (120 ml) heavy cream or plant-based half-and-half

1 cup (240 ml) unsweetened hemp milk or whole milk

½ cup (50 g) freshly grated Parmesan cheese or vegan Parmesan, divided

¼ teaspoon freshly ground black pepper

⅛ teaspoon freshly grated nutmeg

¼ cup (30 g) grated Gruyère cheese or dairy-free shredded cheese

1½ cups (75 g) panko breadcrumbs

30 to 60 mg full-spectrum CBD oil

METHOD OF PREPARATION:

❶ Preheat the oven to 400°F (200°C).

❷ Drain the thawed spinach in a colander in the sink, squeezing out as much liquid as possible. Squeeze the artichokes dry as well. Roughly chop the spinach and artichokes and set both aside.

❸ In medium saucepan over medium heat, heat 2 tablespoons of olive oil.

❹ Add the onion and a pinch of salt. Sweat the onions until translucent, 8 to 10 minutes.

❺ Stir in the flour and cook, stirring, for 2 minutes.

❻ Add the heavy cream and milk and cook until thickened, 2 to 3 minutes.

❼ Add the spinach and artichokes to the sauce and stir until combined.

❽ Add ¼ cup (25 g) of Parmesan cheese and mix well. Season with the remaining salt, the pepper, and nutmeg. Transfer the mixture to a baking dish.

❾ Sprinkle with the remaining ¼ cup (25 g) of Parmesan and the Gruyère. Bake for about 20 minutes, or until lightly browned and bubbly.

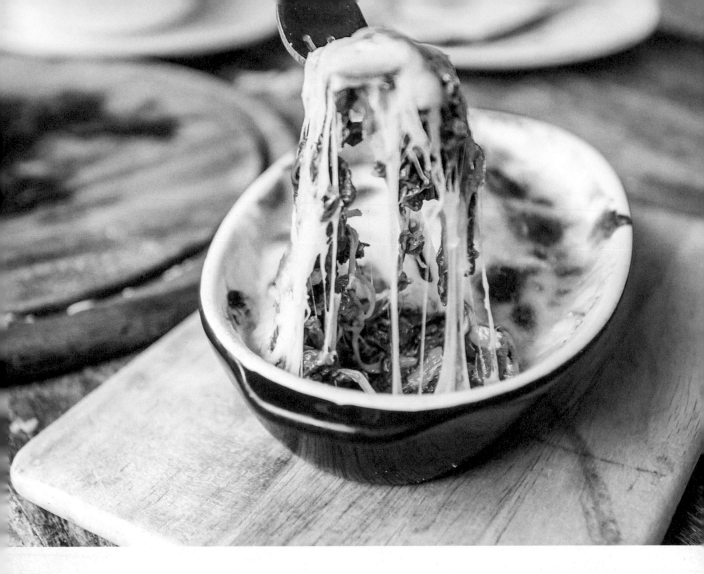

⑩   While the gratin bakes, in a small bowl, stir together the breadcrumbs, remaining 2 tablespoons of olive oil, and CBD oil. Mix well.

⑪   During the last 5 minutes of baking drop the oven temperature to 350° F (180° C) remove the gratin from the oven, sprinkle with the CBD breadcrumbs, and bake for the final 5 minutes. Serve hot!

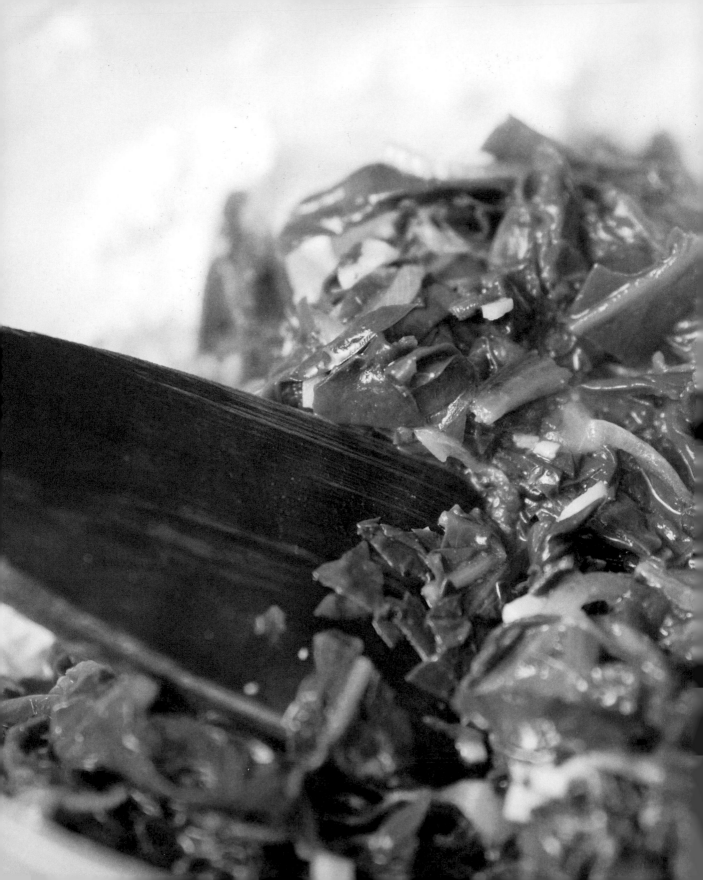

BRAISED WINTER GREENS
WITH BLACK GARLIC & CBD

Yield: Serves 6 / 10 mg per serving

Kale, mustard greens, and escarole are three of my favorite greens, if you prefer spinach and chard then by all means use those, but the combination of cruciferous kale, spicy mustard, and bitter escarole are delicious.

INGREDIENTS

3 tablespoons (45 ml) olive oil
1 medium onion, chopped
1 head black garlic, peeled and sliced
2 pounds (908 g) mix of Tuscan kale, mustard greens, and escarole
1½ cups (360 ml) good-quality vegetable broth
½ cup (120 ml) dry white wine
1½ teaspoons sea salt
1 teaspoon freshly ground black pepper
60 mg full-spectrum CBD oil

TIP *Black garlic is fermented garlic and is quite readily available in most grocery stores. If you cannot find it, you may always use regular chopped garlic.*

METHOD OF PREPARATION:

① In a Dutch oven over medium heat, heat the olive oil until hot. Add the onion and black garlic and cook, stirring frequently, for 4 to 5 minutes, or until softened and beginning to brown.

② Add half the greens and cook, stirring, until they begin to wilt, about 2 minutes.

③ Add the remaining greens to the pot, along with the vegetable broth, wine, salt, and pepper. Bring the mixture to a boil, reduce the heat to low, cover the pot, and simmer for 25 to 30 minutes.

④ Turn off the heat and stir in the CBD oil until well dispersed.

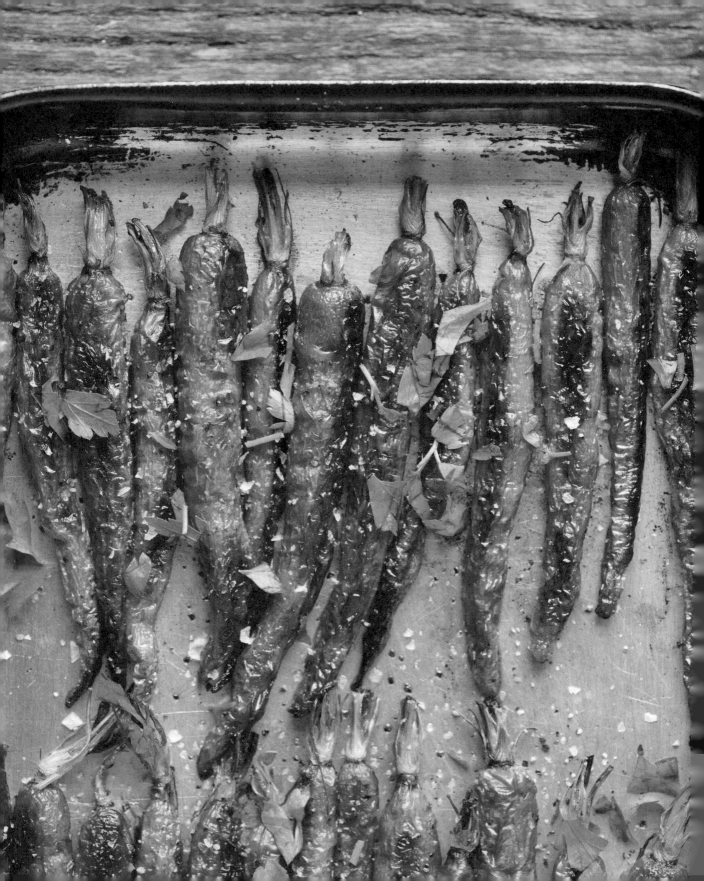

ROASTED GINGER CARROTS
WITH CBD MISO SAUCE

Yield: Serves 8 / 10 to 20 mg per serving

Roasted carrots are so incredibly sweet and complex. Combine them with this miso sauce and you have perfection. This dish has a moderate CBD dose.

INGREDIENTS

2 pounds (908 g) young carrots, peeled and split crosswise

2 tablespoons (30 ml) extra-virgin olive oil

2 garlic cloves, minced

1 tablespoon (6 g) minced, peeled fresh ginger

1½ teaspoons sea salt

¼ cup (60 ml) mirin*

2 tablespoons (34 g) yellow miso paste

2 tablespoons (30 ml) sesame oil

2 tablespoons (30 ml) seasoned rice vinegar

1 tablespoon (15 ml) tamari

80 to 160 mg full-spectrum CBD oil

Mirin can be found in most Asian sections of a grocery store. It is a Japanese sweet rice wine.

METHOD OF PREPARATION:

❶ Preheat the oven to 400°F (200°C). Line a baking sheet with parchment paper.

❷ On the prepared baking sheet, combine the carrots, olive oil, garlic, ginger, and salt. Toss to coat. Roast for about 30 minutes, or until fork-tender and browned on the outside.

❸ While the carrots roast, make the sauce. In a blender, combine the mirin, miso paste, sesame oil, vinegar, tamari, and CBD oil. Purée until smooth.

❹ To serve, arrange the carrots on a platter and pour the sauce over. Serve immediately.

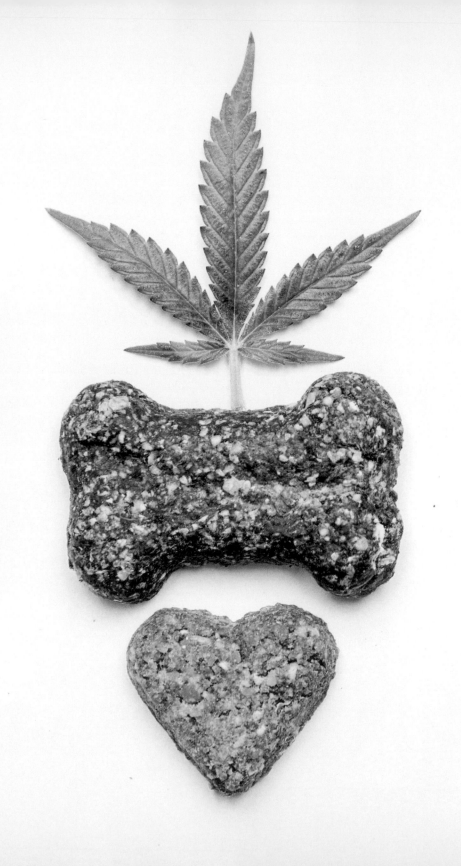

PET SNACKS

BACON-SWEET POTATO
CBD TREATS

Yield: Makes about 36 treats / about 3 mg per treat

My pup loves sweet potato and it is so good for their coat. Mix that with bacon and you have a treat that disappears as quickly as you make them.

INGREDIENTS

2 medium sweet potatoes, scrubbed
12 ounces (340 g) bacon
1½ cups (120 g) quick cooking oats
120 mg full-spectrum CBD oil

METHOD OF PREPARATION:

❶ Preheat the oven to 400°F (200°C). Line two baking sheets with parchment paper.

❷ Place the sweet potatoes on one of the prepared baking sheets and bake for 40 to 50 minutes, or until tender. Set aside to cool. Reserve the parchment-lined sheet.

❸ Reduce the oven temperature to 350°F (180°C).

❹ On the same parchment-lined baking sheet, arrange the bacon in a single layer. Bake for 25 to 30 minutes, flipping halfway through the baking time, until the bacon is crispy. Transfer to a paper towel–lined plate to drain and let cool.

❺ In a food processor, process the cooled bacon until finely chopped. Scrape the bacon out of the food processor and set aside.

❻ Peel the cooled sweet potatoes and place the flesh in a large bowl. Mash well with a fork or potato masher.

❼ Add the bacon, oats, and CBD oil and stir to combine.

❽ Spoon tablespoon-size (15 g) portions onto the second prepared baking sheet. Flatten each to ¼-inch (0.6 cm) thickness.

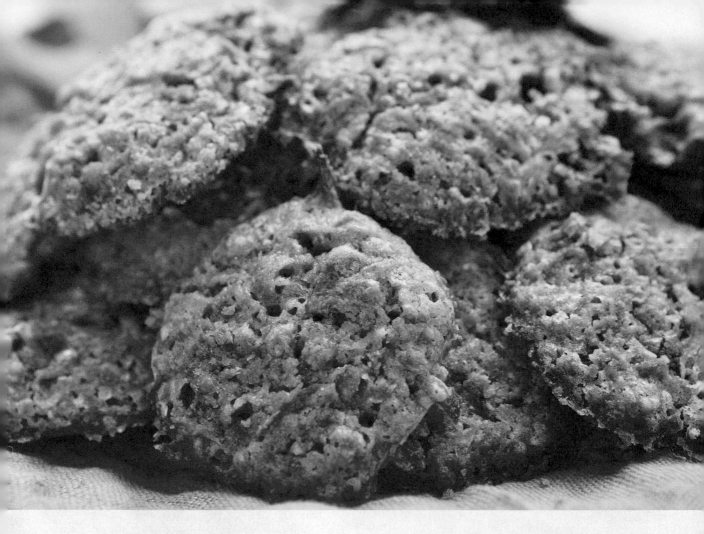

9 Reduce the oven temperature to 225°F (107°C).

10 Bake the treats for 2 to 2½ hours until they are dried out.

11 Cool completely before storing in an airtight container for up to 1 week in the refrigerator.

TIP *Double this recipe and store half in an airtight container in the freezer for later...be warned that they might just disappear too quickly to even freeze!*

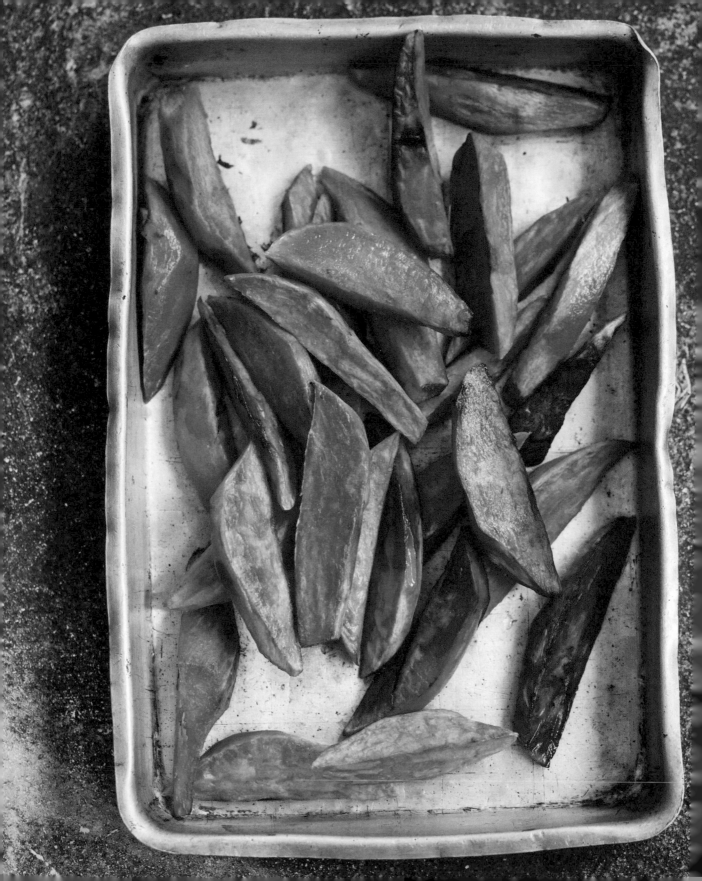

SWEET POTATO & SALMON
CBD CAT TREATS

Yield: Makes about 36 treats / about 3 mg per treat

These kitty treats take a little bit of time, but your feline friend will thank you.

INGREDIENTS

2 sweet potatoes, scrubbed
½ cup (56 g) coconut flour
1 large egg
½ cup (112 g) coconut oil
¼ cup (28 g) gelatin powder
1 (6 ounces, or 170 g) can wild salmon
   or tuna, drained
100 mg full-spectrum CBD oil

TIP *You can always buy canned mashed sweet potato to make these one step easier.*

METHOD OF PREPARATION:

❶ Preheat the oven to 400°F (200°C). Line a baking sheet with parchment paper.

❷ Place the sweet potatoes on the prepared baking sheet and bake for 40 to 50 minutes, or until tender. Set aside to cool. Set aside the parchment-lined baking sheet for later use. Once cooled, peel the sweet potatoes.

❸ Reduce the oven temperature to 350°F (180°C).

❹ In a large bowl, combine the peeled sweet potatoes with the remaining ingredients. Using a fork, mash everything together until well combined. The dough should be thick and sticky.

❺ Roll the mixture into 1-inch (2.5 cm) balls and place on the reserved baking sheet. Mash down each ball with a fork.

❻ Bake for 20 minutes, or until lightly browned.

❼ Cool completely before refrigerating in an airtight container for several weeks, or freezing for several months.

MACKEREL & COCONUT
CBD CAT TREATS

Yield: Makes about 18 treats / about 3 mg per treat

Cats need CBD too! These fishy treats are simple and a delicious way to calm that furry friend.

INGREDIENTS

½ cup (95 g) canned mackerel, drained
    and crumbled
1 cup (115 g) whole-grain breadcrumbs
1 tablespoon (14 g) coconut oil
50 mg full-spectrum CBD oil
1 large egg, beaten
½ teaspoon brewer's yeast

METHOD OF PREPARATION:

❶ Preheat the oven to 350°F (180°C). Line a baking sheet with parchment paper and set aside.

❷ In a large bowl, combine all the ingredients and mix well. Drop ¼-teaspoonful amounts onto the prepared baking sheet, 1 inch (2.5 cm) apart.

❸ Bake for 8 minutes until they are and lightly browned.

❹ Let cool completely before refrigerating in an airtight container for up to 1 week.

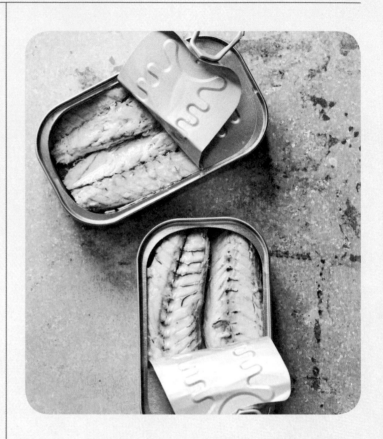

TIP *Do NOT swap tuna for the canned mackerel in these treats. You need the oily fish to make these work.*

TUNA CBD THUMBPRINT
CAT TREATS

Yield: Makes 24 treats / 4 mg per treat

Get your cat to love you (or at least acknowledge that you exist) with these simple, homemade treats.

INGREDIENTS

5 ounces (140 g) canned tuna, drained and flaked
½ cup (70 g) cornmeal
½ cup (79 g) brown rice flour
½ cup (120 ml) water
75 mg full-spectrum CBD oil

METHOD OF PREPARATION:

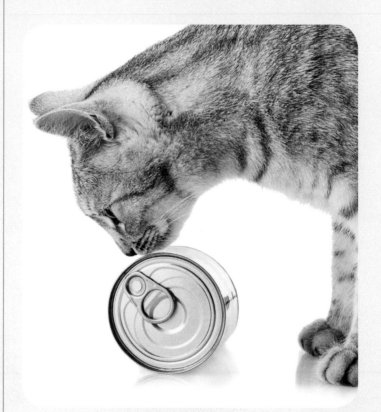

❶ Preheat the oven to 350°F (180°C). Line a baking sheet with parchment paper and set aside.

❷ In a large bowl, stir together all the ingredients until well combined. Break off a tiny piece of the mixture and roll it into a small bite-size treat. Place it on the prepared baking sheet and repeat with the remaining dough.

❸ Flatten each ball with your thumb or a fork.

❹ Bake for 5 minutes. Flip the treats and bake for 5 minutes more until dried and lightly browned.

❺ Let cool completely before refrigerating in an airtight container for up to 1 week.

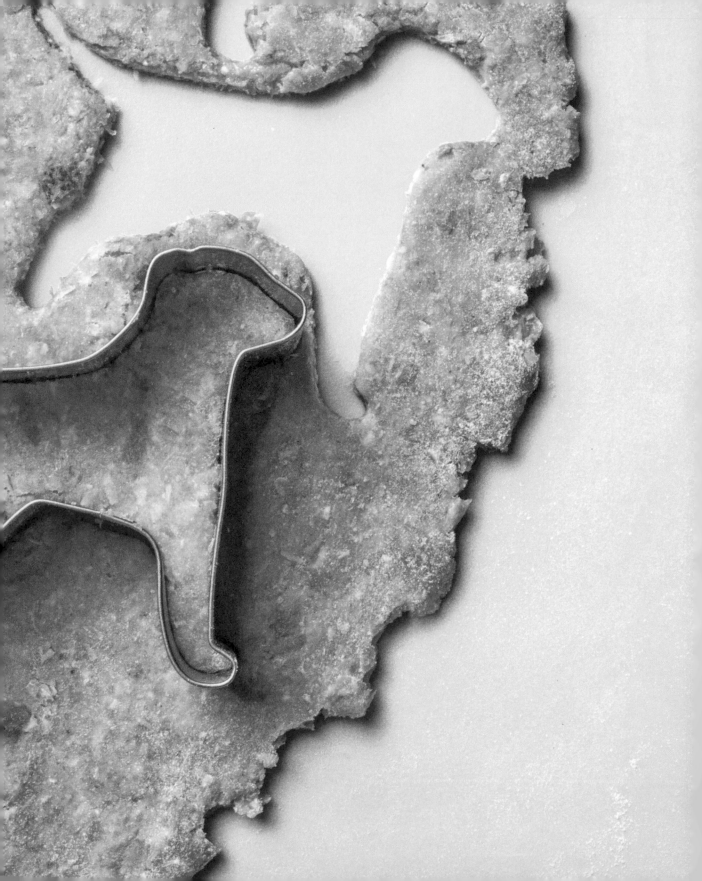

YUMMY CBD
DOG TREATS

Yield: Makes 30 treats / 4 mg per treat

These could not be simpler, and my pup loves them! Play around and get creative with types of baby food.

INGREDIENTS

4 (2.5 ounces, or 71 g each) jars baby food—puréed meat or vegetables or a combination
2 cups (316 g) brown rice flour, plus more for the work surface
1 cup (156 g) old-fashioned rolled oats
1 cup (112 g) wheat germ
120 mg full-spectrum CBD oil

TIP *Keep some extra jars of baby food on hand to whip these treats up for your beloved pup!*

METHOD OF PREPARATION:

1. Preheat the oven to 350°F (180°C). Line a baking sheet with parchment paper and set aside.

2. In a large bowl, stir together all the treat ingredients to form a dough.

3. Lightly flour a work surface and turn the dough out on to it. Roll out the dough to ¼-inch (0.6 cm) thickness and cut it into desired shapes.

4. Transfer the cutouts to the prepared baking sheet and bake for 20 to 25 minutes. Turn off the oven and leave the baking sheet inside the oven until the oven is completely cool.

5. Store the treats in an airtight container for up to 1 week.

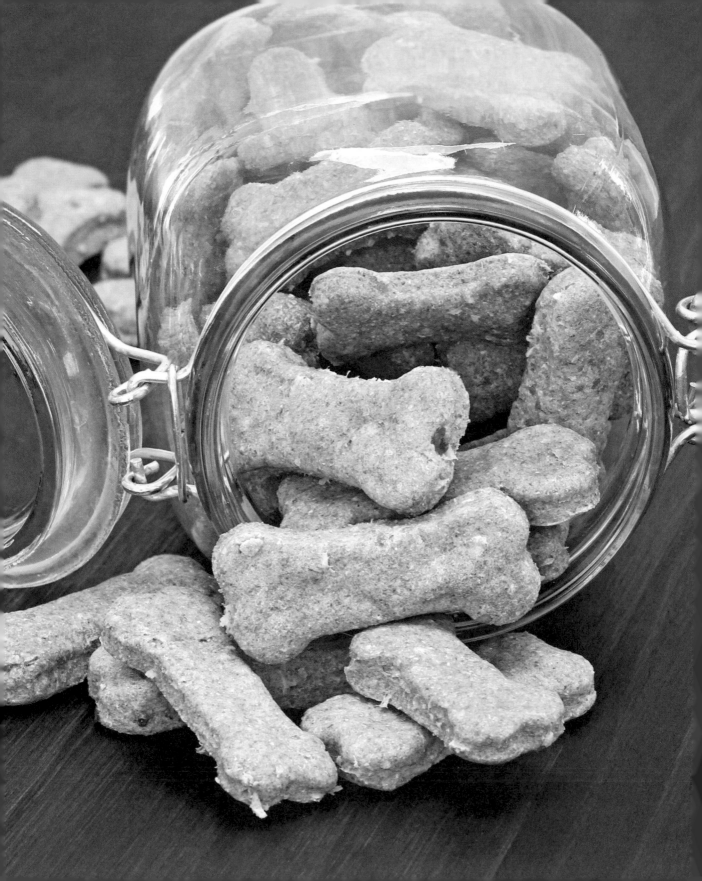

GINGER-APPLE
CBD BONES

Yield: Makes 25 bones / 4 mg per treat

These are great for when your pup has a little bit of an upset stomach. Ginger is a natural tummy tamer, and combine that with the calming CBD and you have a great way to soothe your pup.

INGREDIENTS

1 cup (158 g) brown rice flour
½ cup (75 g) finely diced peeled apple
⅔ cup (153 g) plain nonfat Greek yogurt
½ teaspoon ground ginger
1 tablespoon (14 g) coconut oil
100 mg full-spectrum CBD oil

METHOD OF PREPARATION:

1. Preheat the oven to 350°F (180°C). Line a baking sheet with parchment paper and set aside.

2. In a large bowl, stir together all the ingredients until well mixed.

3. Lightly flour a work surface and turn the mixture out on to it. Roll it out to ¼-inch (0.6 cm) thickness and cut out shapes with a bone cookie cutter or any other desired shape. Transfer the cutouts to the prepared baking sheet.

4. Bake for 25 minutes, or until golden brown.

5. Let cool completely before storing in an airtight container for up to 1 week.

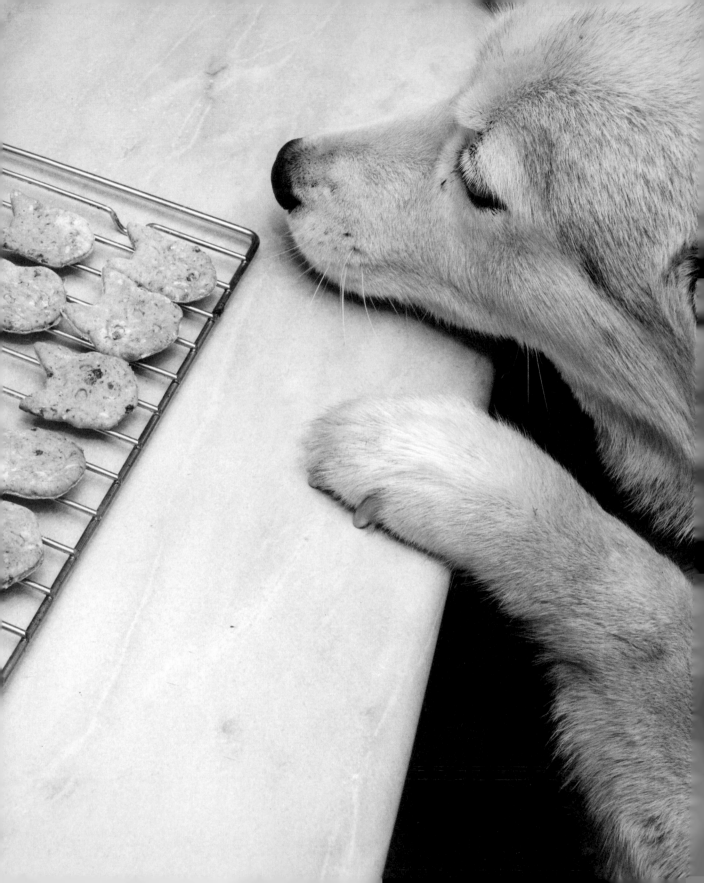

CBD HONEY & PEANUT BUTTER
DOG BISCUITS

Yield: Makes 12 biscuits / 4 mg per biscuit

These are a huge hit in my house! The combination of honey and peanut butter seem to be a home run for my pup.

INGREDIENTS

1 tablespoon (14 g) coconut oil
50 mg full-spectrum CBD oil
1 cup (240 ml) chicken broth
½ cup (130 g) peanut butter
¼ cup (80 g) honey
1 cup (156 g) old-fashioned rolled oats
1 cup (125 g) whole-wheat flour
1 cup (124 g) all-purpose flour, plus more
   for the work surface

TIP *These can be made and frozen for up to 1 month in an airtight container.*

METHOD OF PREPARATION:

1. Preheat the oven to 350°F (180°C). Line a baking sheet with parchment paper and set aside.

2. In a large bowl, whisk the coconut oil, CBD oil, chicken broth, peanut butter, and honey.

3. Add the dry ingredients to the wet ingredients and stir until thoroughly combined. Lightly flour a work surface and turn the dough out on to it. Roll out the dough to ¼-inch (0.6 cm) thickness.

4. Using a cookie cutter (I love a bone shape, but you can use a circle shape if that's what you have) cut out cookie shapes and place them on the prepared baking sheet.

5. Bake for 14 to 16 minutes until dry and lightly browned. Let the treats cool completely before removing from the baking sheet. Store in an airtight container for up to 2 weeks.

COCONUT AND TURMERIC
CBD BREATH MINTS

Yield: Makes 20 mints / 4 mg per treat

What dog doesn't need the occasional breath mint? Mine sure does! These are a great combination of mint and an anxiety reducer.

INGREDIENTS

1½ cups (336 g) coconut oil
80 mg full-spectrum CBD oil
1 cup (60 g) fresh parsley, chopped
½ cup (48 g) fresh mint, chopped
1 teaspoon ground turmeric

METHOD OF PREPARATION:

1. Line a baking sheet with parchment paper and set aside.

2. In a large microwave-safe bowl, microwave the coconut oil on high power for about 30 seconds, or just until softened.

3. Stir in the CBD oil, parsley, mint, and turmeric, mixing well.

4. Roll the mixture into 1-inch (2.5 cm) balls and place them on the prepared baking sheet. Alternatively, pour the mixture into a silicone mold.

5. Refrigerate for at least 1 hour. Keep the mints refrigerated in an airtight container for up to two weeks.

FROZEN PEANUT BUTTER
YOGURT TREATS

Yield: Makes 24 treats / 5 mg per treat

Dogs need some cool summer treats just like we do. I make a batch of these on those hot summer days and my pup gobbles them up.

INGREDIENTS

1 cup (260 g) creamy peanut butter, melted

1 quart (960 g) plain nonfat yogurt

120 mg full-spectrum CBD oil

METHOD OF PREPARATION:

❶ Line 2 rimmed baking sheets with parchment paper and set aside.

❷ In a large bowl, whisk the melted peanut butter, yogurt, and CBD oil until smooth.

❸ Using a medium cookie scoop, drop mounds of the peanut butter mixture onto the prepared baking sheets. Freeze for 1 hour, or until completely frozen. Transfer the treats to a freezer-safe container or zipper bag and keep frozen for up to 2 months.

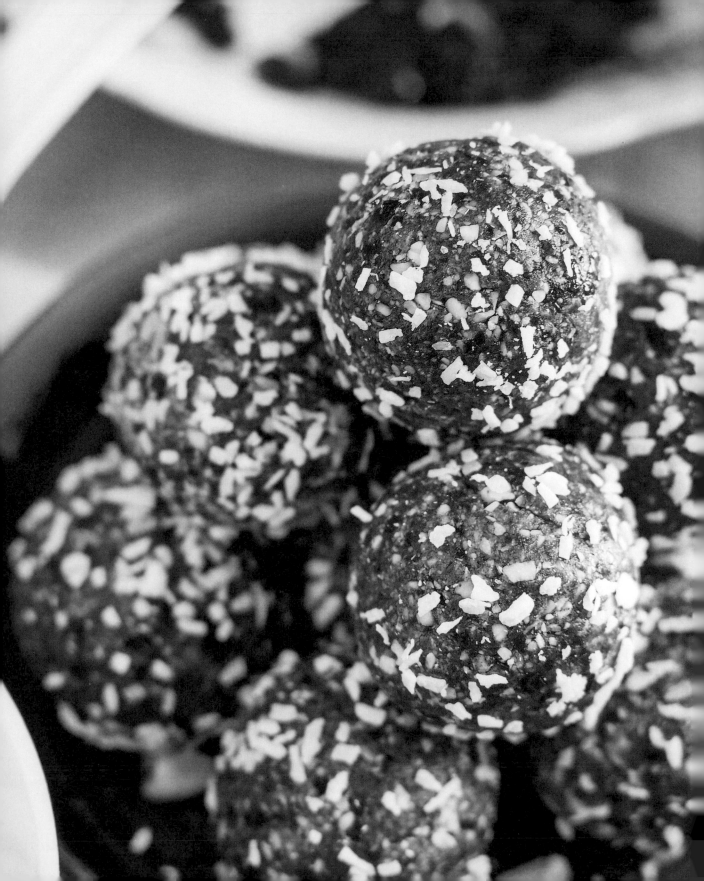

NO-BAKE COCONUT OAT BALL
DOG TREATS

Yield: Makes 36 balls / 5 mg per treat

These easy no bake treats are a crowd pleaser for all dogs. I doubled the recipe and froze them for up to one month... that's how easy they are.

INGREDIENTS

⅔ cup (53 g) finely shredded unsweetened coconut
⅔ cup (149 g) coconut oil
180 mg full-spectrum CBD oil
6 tablespoons (96 g) creamy peanut butter
5 cups (780 g) old-fashioned rolled oats

 TIP *These are so good, even your pup's human will love them!*

METHOD OF PREPARATION:

❶ Place the shredded coconut in a small bowl and set aside.

❷ In a food processor, process the coconut oil, CBD oil, peanut butter and rolled oats until smooth. Scoop out tablespoon-size (14 g) pieces and roll into balls.

❸ Toss the balls gently in the shredded coconut and place them on a rimmed baking sheet.

❹ Refrigerate for 30 minutes, or until set. Keep refrigerated in an airtight container for up to 1 week.

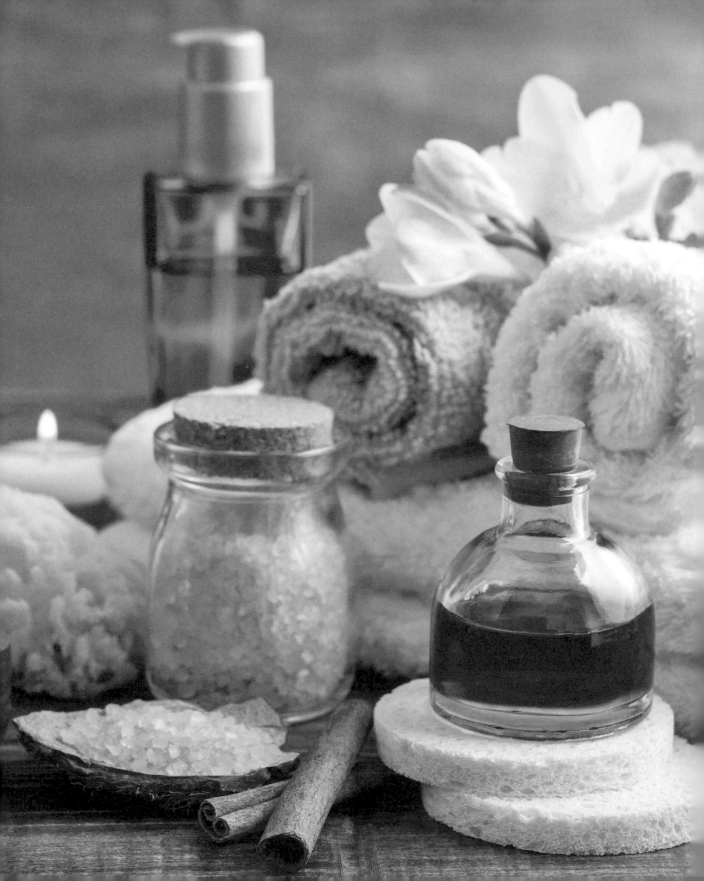

SELF-CARE

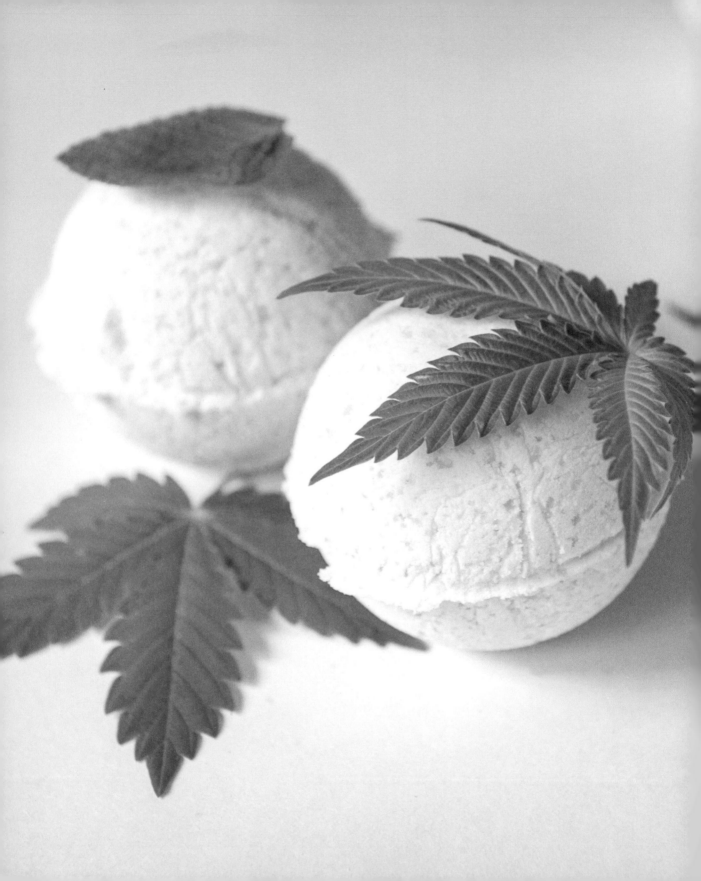

ESSENTIAL OIL
CBD BATH BOMBS

Yield: Makes 1 bath bomb

There is not much that a hot bath does not cure. This CBD-infused bath bomb will relax you to the core. Play around with the essential oils and create your ultimate bath experience.

INGREDIENTS

Bath bomb molds
4 ounces (115 g) baking soda
2 ounces (55 g) cornstarch
2 ounces (55 g) citric acid
2 ounces (55 g) Epsom salts
1½ teaspoons water, plus more as needed
1 teaspoon essential oil of choice
¼ teaspoon CBD-infused coconut oil
3 drops food coloring of choice (optional)

TIP *If you cannot find CBD-infused coconut oil, simply add 25 mg of CBD isolate to the recipe and use ¼ teaspoon of regular coconut oil.*

METHOD OF PREPARATION:

1. In a bowl, combine all the dry ingredients and whisk until evenly mixed.

2. In a shot glass, combine the wet ingredients, including the food coloring (if using). Very slowly, whisk the liquid mixture into the dry mixture. If it fizzes, you are going too fast.

3. Very slowly, whisk the liquid mixture into the dry mixture. If it fizzes, you are going too fast and need to slow down. Once the ingredients are evenly combined, the mixture will resemble damp sand. The mixture should stick together when squeezed. Add more water if it doesn't stick together.

4. Fill the mold halves with the mixture until they are a little over filled. Do not pack too densely. Loosely sprinkle some more of the mixture on each half to help the two stick together. Press the two halves together firmly and hold for a few seconds. Gently remove one side of the mold.

5. Set the bath bomb down, mold-side down, and let dry for 20 minutes.

6. Using a gentle twisting motion, carefully remove the other side of the mold. Let sit for a few hours, or overnight, until the bath bomb is totally firm.

7. Drop into your bath when ready to relax.

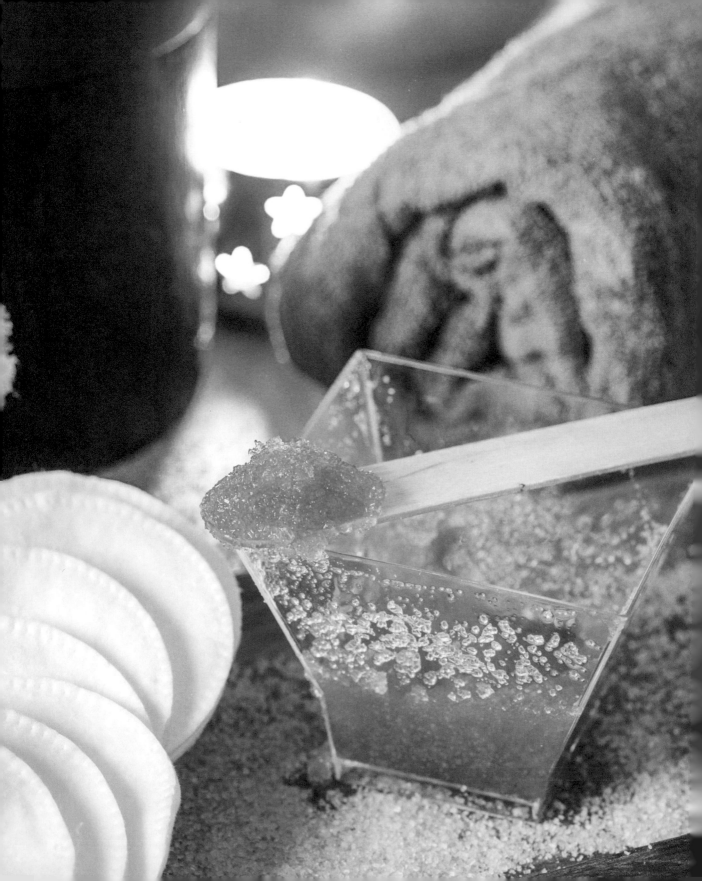

CBD BROWN SUGAR SCRUB
WITH AVOCADO & HONEY

Yield: Makes 1 cup

This scrub is divine! It smells scrumptious, leaves your body feeling smooth and has the added benefit of relieving sore muscles.

INGREDIENTS

0.5 g CBD isolate
2 tablespoons (30 ml) avocado oil
2 tablespoons (30 ml) olive oil
½ cup (160 g) Manuka honey
1 cup (225 g) packed organic brown sugar
2 tablespoons (12 g) orange zest
Few drops quality grade peppermint or lavender essential oil

TIP *Use high-quality ingredients, organic if possible. This is going on your skin, which is just as important as what goes into your body.*

METHOD OF PREPARATION:

1. In a medium bowl, whisk the CBD isolate, avocado oil, and olive oil.

2. Add the honey and whisk to combine.

3. Stir in the brown sugar, orange zest, and essential oil.

4. To use, warm and thoroughly wet skin in a shower with warm water. Apply scrub with hands and massage into skin. Wash off thoroughly.

5. Store leftovers in a Mason jar for up to 6 months.

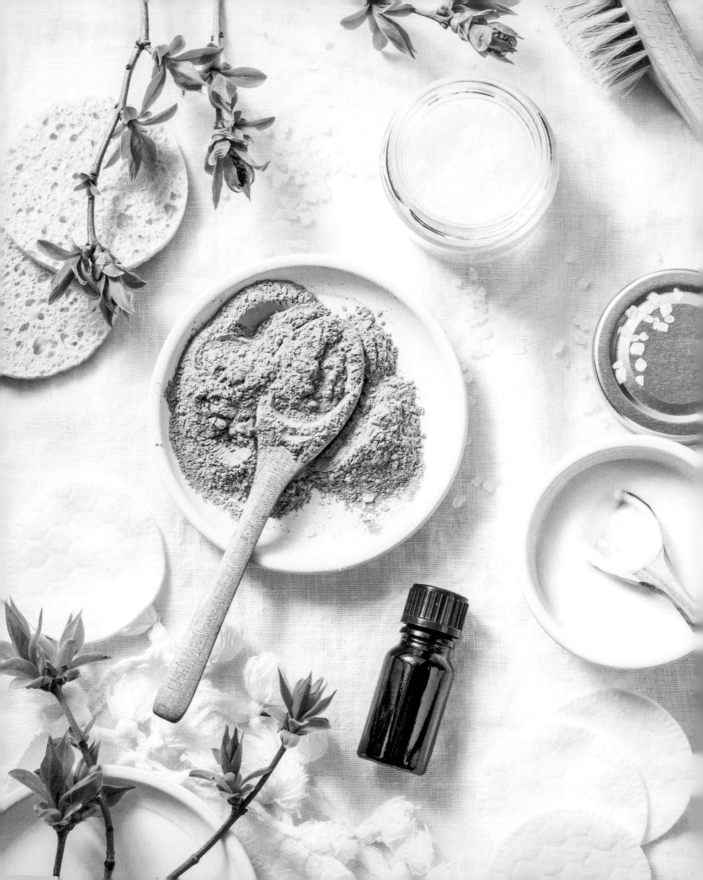

CBD FACE MASK
FOR OILY SKIN

Yield: Makes enough for 1 application

CBD has been shown to help with reducing the bacteria that causes acne. This mask is twofold. It helps fight the oil and helps reduce the bacteria that causes acne.

INGREDIENTS

1½ teaspoons bentonite clay
1 teaspoon Manuka honey
1 teaspoon organic apple cider vinegar
1 g CBD isolate

TIP *Bentonite clay is an absorbent kind of clay that typically forms after volcanic clay ages. This clay has a unique composition and can absorb "negatively charged" toxins.*

METHOD OF PREPARATION:

1. In a small wooden, glass, or ceramic bowl, combine all the mask ingredients and mix well.

2. Apply to clean dry skin. Wait until the clay begins to harden and crack, about 15 to 20 minutes, before gently removing the mask with warm water and a washcloth.

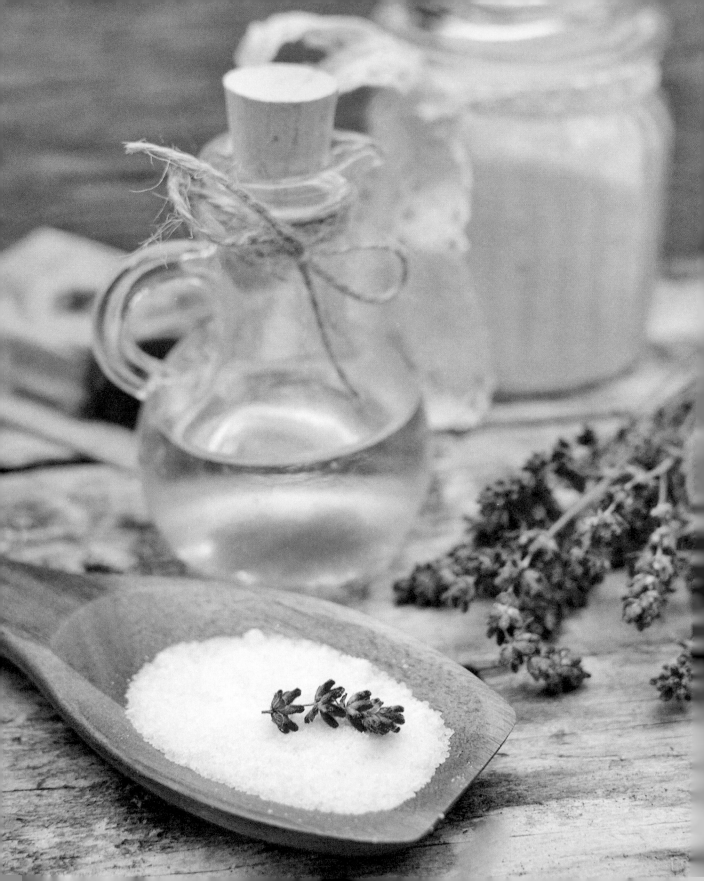

CBD FOOT SOAK
WITH TEA TREE & PEPPERMINT OILS

Yield: Makes enough for 4 soaks

If you stand on your feet all day long, this soak is for you. This will leave your feet feeling invigorated and so refreshed.

INGREDIENTS

1 cup (249 g) Epsom salts
2 tablespoons (30 ml) full-spectrum CBD oil
6 drops tea tree essential oil
6 drops peppermint essential oil

TIP *Epsom salts are not actually a salt, but a naturally occurring pure mineral compound of magnesium and sulfate. That's why it is so amazing for sore muscles.*

METHOD OF PREPARATION:

1. In a medium glass bowl, combine all the foot soak ingredients and mix well.

2. Fill your foot soak tub with warm water and add ¼ cup of the mixture. Soak your feet for 20 minutes, or until you're ultimately relaxed.

3. Store the remaining foot soak in a Mason jar in a dark dry spot for up to 3 months.

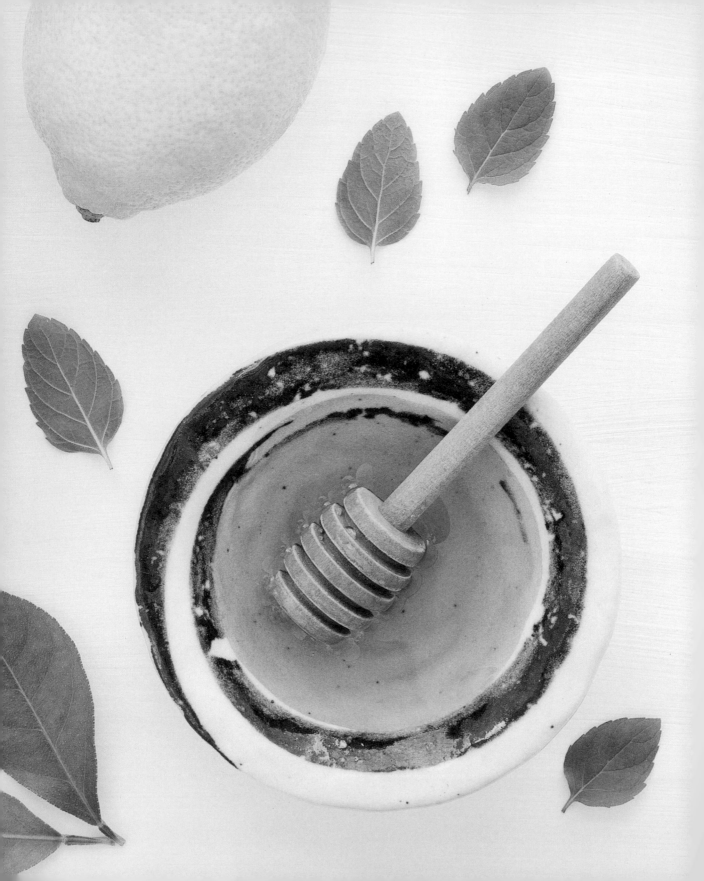

CBD ANTI-INFLAMMATION MASK
WITH LEMON, HONEY & TURMERIC

Yield: Makes enough for 1 application

CBD, manuka honey, turmeric, and apple cider vinegar. This mask is chock full of antibacterial, antimicrobial, anti-inflammatory, exfoliating powerhouses! This mask will leave your skin glowing.

INGREDIENTS

2 tablespoons (30 ml) fresh lemon juice
1 tablespoon (20 g) Manuka honey
1 teaspoon full-spectrum CBD oil
½ teaspoon ground turmeric
½ teaspoon hemp milk
½ teaspoon extra-virgin olive oil
½ teaspoon organic apple cider vinegar

TIP *Turmeric can stain pale skin. If this happens, soak a cotton ball in coconut or castor oil, dab it over the stained skin and voila!*

METHOD OF PREPARATION:

1. In a small bowl, stir together all the mask ingredients.

2. Apply to a clean face, avoiding the eyes and lips.

3. Leave on for 20 to 30 minutes. Wash off and love how your skin feels!

CBD PEPPERMINT
FOOT EXFOLIATION SCRUB

Yield: Makes 1 cup, enough for about 8 applications

This is by far my favorite DIY product. To any person with exhausted feet, this is for you. The combination of tea tree and peppermint oil with CBD will leave your feet feeling tingly and alive.

INGREDIENTS

1 cup (236 g) sea salt
1 tablespoon (15 ml) olive oil
1 tablespoon (14 g) coconut oil, melted but not hot
5 drops tea tree essential oil
5 drops peppermint essential oil
5 drops lavender essential oil
300 mg full-spectrum CBD oil or 3 g CBD isolate

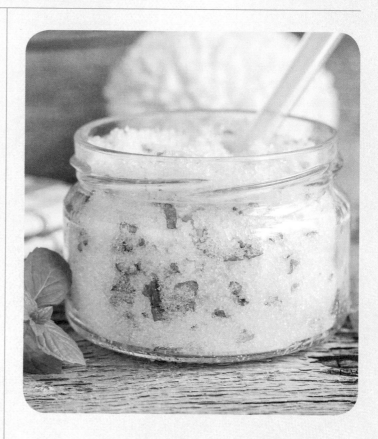

MEHOD OF PREPARATION:

1. Place the sea salt in a medium glass bowl. Stir in the olive oil and coconut oil until well blended.

2. Add the essential oils and CBD of choice and blend to combine all ingredients.

3. Store in a Mason jar for up to 6 months and use whenever your feet need a little extra love.

CBD PEPPERMINT
LIP BALM

Yield: Makes 3 tubes

*Have you ever made your own lip balm?
Me either! But after making this one,
I am hooked. This calming and tingly
balm is incredible for healing chapped
lips or just bringing a little life back
into tired ones.*

INGREDIENTS

1½ teaspoons beeswax
2 teaspoons avocado butter
2 teaspoons full-spectrum CBD oil
3 drops peppermint essential oil

METHOD OF PREPARATION:

❶   In a double boiler over medium
heat, combine the beeswax and
avocado butter. Cook, stirring
occasionally, until the mixture
melts.

❷   Turn off the heat and whisk in
the CBD oil and peppermint oil.
Working quickly and carefully,
pour the mixture into the lip balm
containers.

❸   Let the lip balm cool for 20
minutes. Store in a cool dry place.

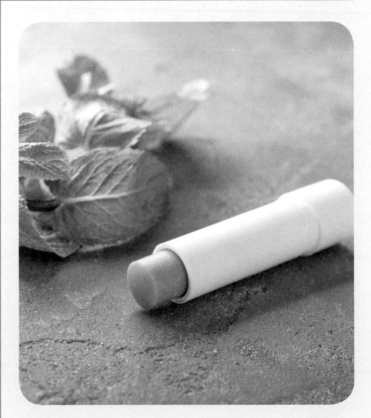

TIP   *Both lip balm tubes and beeswax are easily
found online or at craft stores.*

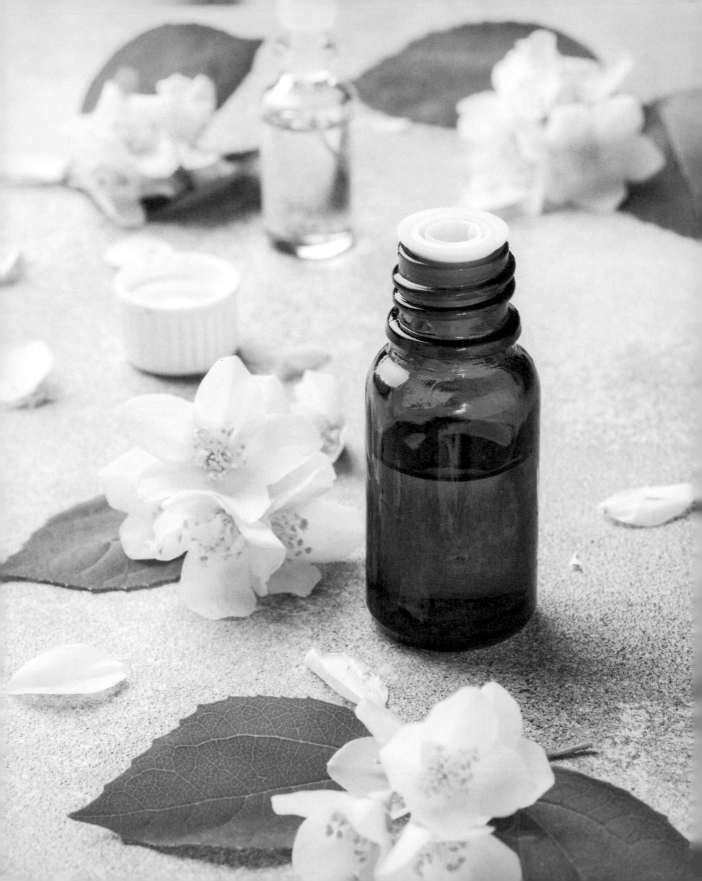

CBD PMS BATH BLEND
WITH ALMOND, BERGAMOT & SAGE

Yield: Makes enough for 1 bath

A bath is my favorite way to send a little healing to my body during my cycle. This bath blend rejuvenates the body and aids in the healing process that is needed as a woman. Light some candles, turn out the lights and allow this bath soak to work its magic.

INGREDIENTS

20 to 40 mg full-spectrum CBD oil
1 tablespoon (15 ml) sweet almond oil
4 drops bergamot essential oil
4 drops clary sage essential oil
2 drops geranium essential oil
1 drop ylang-ylang essential oil

METHOD OF PREPARATION:

❶ In a small wooden, glass, or ceramic bowl, combine all the oils.

❷ Add them to your warm bath and soak for 15 to 30 minutes.

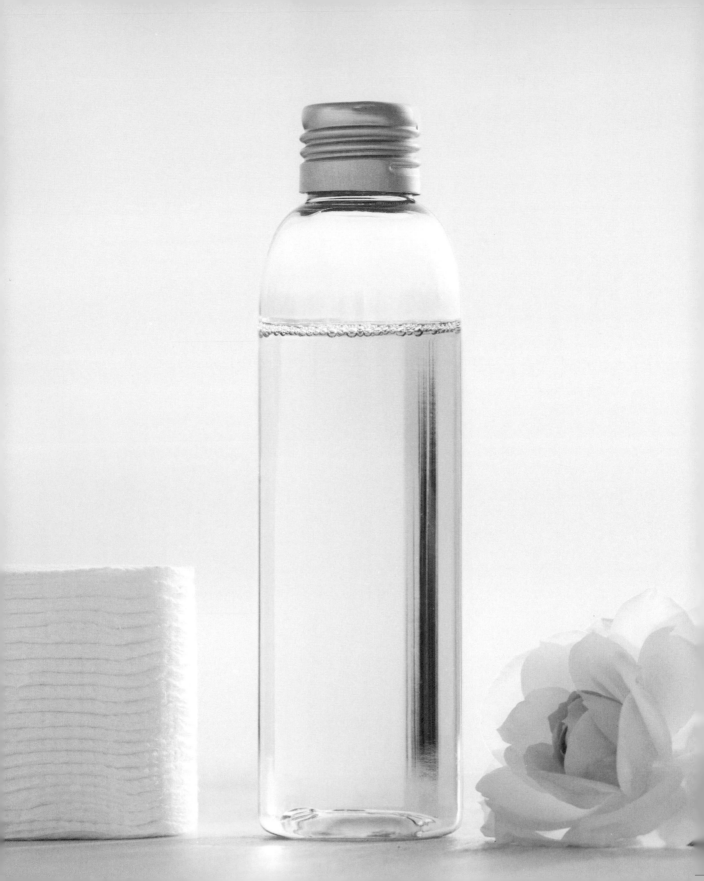

ROSE-LAVENDER
CBD FACIAL TONER

Yield: Makes about 4 ounces (120 ml)

A toner is a great vehicle to deliver and correct the pH balance of the skin, especially for acne-prone skin. This one has a calming anti-inflammatory property.

INGREDIENTS

2 ounces (60 ml) rose flower water
1 ounce (30 ml) witch hazel extract
1 tablespoon (15 ml) aloe vera gel
½ teaspoon vegetable glycerin
7 drops lavender essential oil
4 drops chamomile extract
100 mg full-spectrum CBD oil

TIP *This makes an incredibly beautiful gift. Put toner in a glass jar with a couple of organic rose petals and you have a perfect and thoughtful gift for friends.*

METHOD OF PREPARATION:

1. In a clean 4-ounce (120 ml) glass mister bottle, combine all the toner ingredients. Top with a mister and shake to blend. Keep the toner refrigerated for up to 6 months. Shake a little before each use.

2. To use, wash your face and gently pat dry. Mist your clean face with the toner and let air-dry before applying the remainder of your skin care regimen.

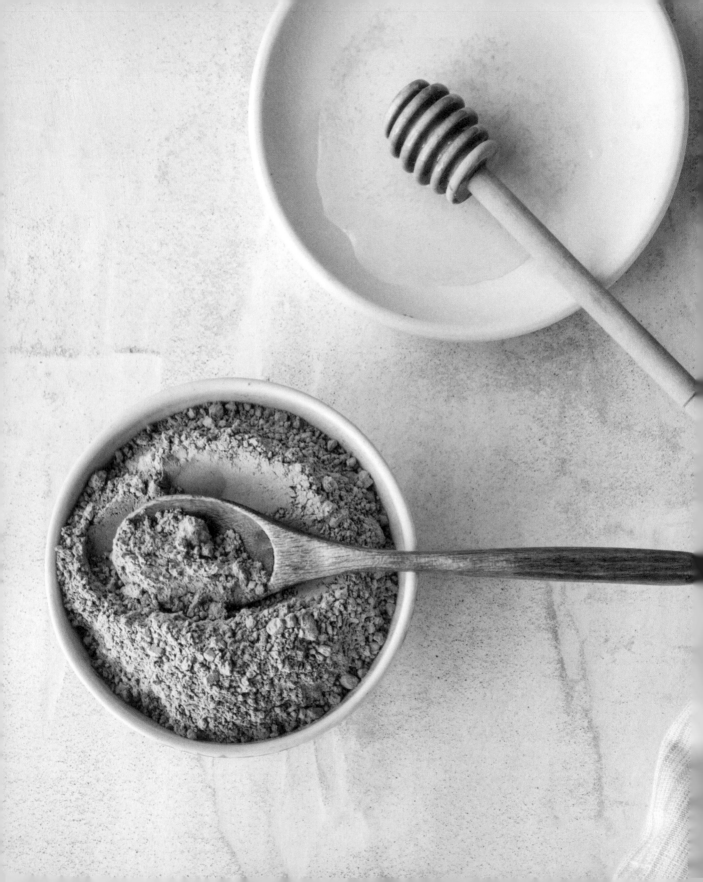

CBD FACE MASK
FOR SENSITIVE SKIN

Yield: Makes enough for 1 application

Manuka honey is a natural anti-microbial/anti-bacterial agent. Matcha powder has many anti-inflammatory properties that help reduce the redness associated with chronic skin conditions such as rosacea acne. These two ingredients together help create a super gentle and loving mask for sensitive skin.

INGREDIENTS

1 teaspoon organic ceremonial-grade
    matcha powder
1 teaspoon Manuka honey
1 teaspoon organic sweet almond oil
1 g CBD isolate

METHOD OF PREPARATION:

❶ In a small wooden, glass, or ceramic bowl, combine all the face mask ingredients and mix well.

❷ Apply to clean dry skin. Relax for 20 minutes. Wipe off with warm water and a washcloth.

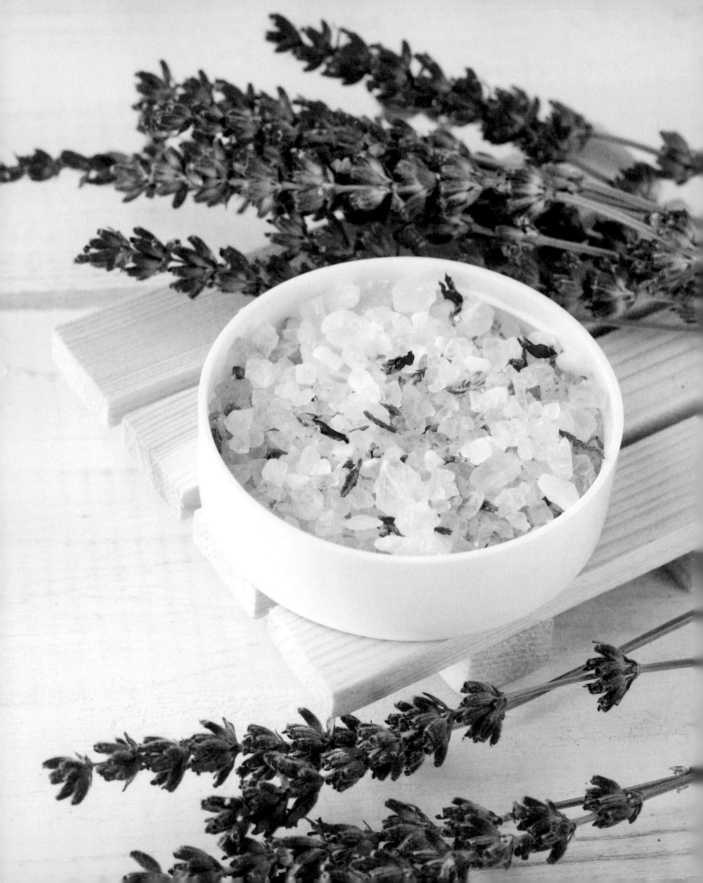

CBD STRESS-RELIEF
EPSOM SALTS WITH LAVENDAR

Yield: Makes enough for 1 bath

Epsom salts have been around to soak tired muscles for a very long time. They are also an incredible source of magnesium, which a wonderful sleep regulator. That combined with CBD make these bath salts the perfect way to wind down and have a blissful night of sleep.

INGREDIENTS

2 cups (499 g) Epsom salts
20 mg CBD isolate
7 drops lavender essential oil
2 drops rose geranium essential oil

TIP *Rose geranium essential oil has an earthy and herbaceous aroma and it is said to have soothing and sedative effects that promote relaxation, emotional stability, and optimism. Sign me up!*

METHOD OF PREPARATION:

❶ In a large glass jar, stir together all the ingredients.

❷ When ready to take a bath, fill the tub with warm water and add the salt soak. Step in and relax.

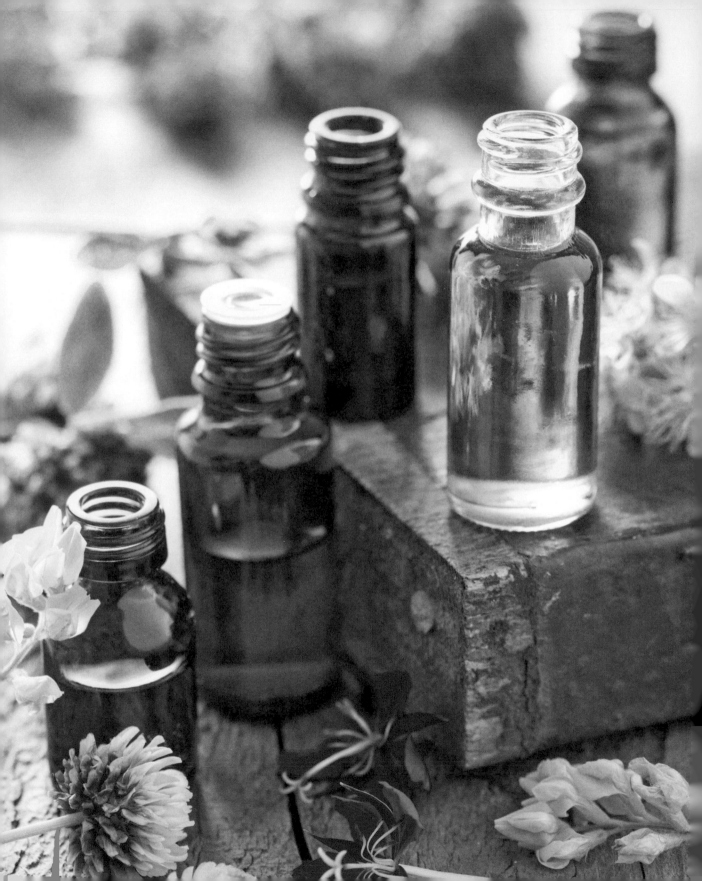

ENERGIZING CBD MASSAGE OIL
WITH ALMOND & JUNIPER BERRY

Yield: Makes about ⅓ cup

The combination of invigorating essential oils and CBD make this massage oil such a delight for sore, tired muscles.

INGREDIENTS

8 drops ginger essential oil
5 drops grapefruit essential oil
3 drops juniper berry essential oil
¼ cup (60 ml) organic sweet almond oil
100 mg full-spectrum CBD oil

TIP *Juniper berry is known as a natural antiseptic and helps alleviate muscle pain. It has even been shown to support kidney and urinary tract function.*

METHOD OF PREPARATION:

1. In a small dark glass bottle, combine all the massage oil ingredients. Cover and shake until blended.

2. Apply liberally.

3. Store in a cool dark place for up to 1 year.

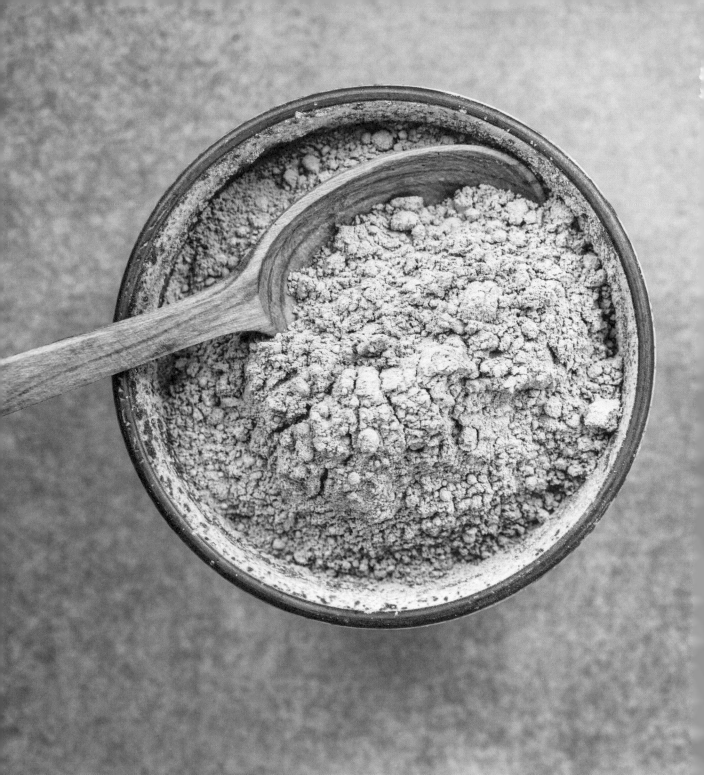

CBD PEPPERMINT MATCHA
CLAY FACE MASK

Yield: Makes enough for 1 application

This mask is so well rounded. The clay helps rid the skin of toxins and impurities, the matcha powder is packed with antioxidants that give your skin a healthy smooth glow, the peppermint is invigorating, and the CBD has anti-inflammatory properties. Honestly, this mask does it all!

INGREDIENTS

2 tablespoons (15 g) white kaolin clay
1 tablespoon (20 g) Manuka honey
¼ teaspoon organic ceremonial-grade
    matcha powder
1 drop peppermint essential oil
20 mg full-spectrum CBD oil
2 teaspoons organic rose water

METHOD OF PREPARATION:

❶   In a small wooden, ceramic, or glass bowl and using a wooden or glass spoon, stir together the clay, honey, matcha, peppermint oil, and CBD oil.

❷   Slowly stir in the rose water until you reach the desired consistency.

❸   Evenly spread the mask over your face, avoiding the mouth and eyes. Leave on for 15 to 20 minutes.

❹   Wash off with warm water and gently pat the skin dry. Follow with your usual skin care regimen.

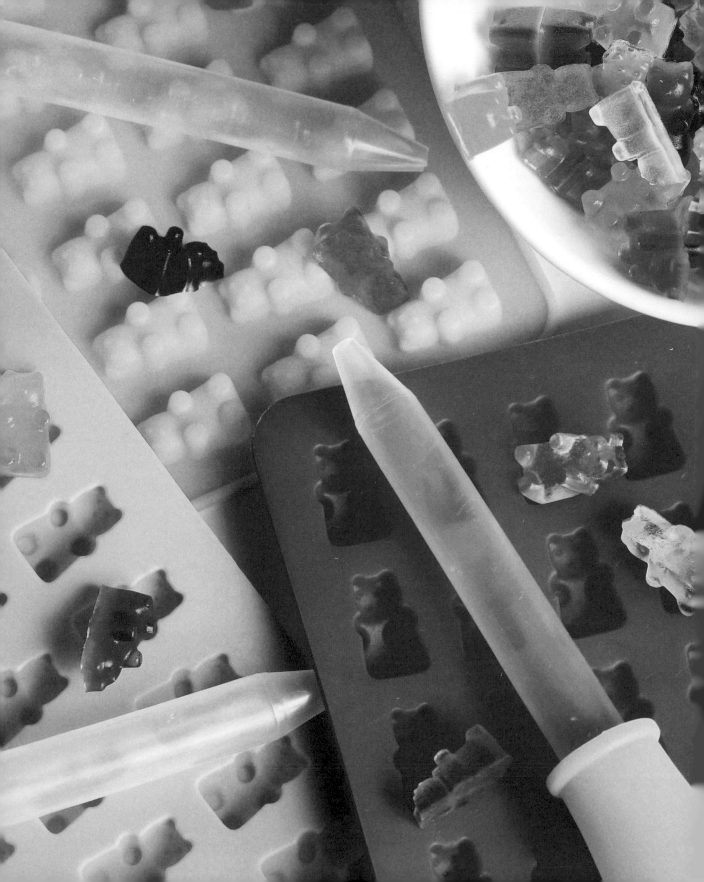

CBD GUMMY BEARS
WITH PEACH, PEAR & LEMON JUICES

Yield: Makes 50 gummy bear–size gummies / 10 mg each

Homemade gummy treats?! These are so simple and such an easy bedtime treat for a great night's rest. Always start with one gummy and see how it makes you feel, increase as needed.

INGREDIENTS

Gummy bear silicone molds
1 cup (240 ml) organic peach juice or pear juice
1 tablespoon (15 ml) fresh lemon juice
2 tablespoons (40 g) raw local honey
3 tablespoons (21 g) organic grass-fed unflavored gelatin
500 mg CBD isolate

TIP *You can easily find any shape gummy mold online. If you don't feel like a bear, make it a lemon or a pineapple ring or even a star.*

METHOD OF PREPARATION:

❶ Place the gummy bear silicone molds on a baking sheet and set aside.

❷ In a medium saucepan over medium-low heat, combine the peach juice, lemon juice, and honey.

❸ Slowly whisk in the gelatin, stirring constantly to avoid clumping. Cook, whisking continually, until all the gelatin is completely melted and incorporated.

❹ Whisk in the CBD isolate until fully dispersed. Turn off the heat.

❺ Pour the mixture into the silicone molds. Use the baking sheet to transfer the molds to the freezer and freeze for 30 minutes.

❻ Remove the molds from the freezer and pop out each gummy. Store them in an airtight container in a cool dark place for up to three weeks.

INDEX